Keto Diet

Table of Contents

Introduction 1

Chapter One: Ketogenic Diet Basics 3

Chapter Two: Understanding the Keto Diet 33

Chapter Three: Benefits of Keto Diet... 37

Chapter Four: Basics of Planning Meals....................................... 45

Chapter Five: Setting up a Plan.. 65

Conclusion 101

Preview Of Intermittent fasting: Beginners Guide To Weight Loss For Men And Women With Intermittent Fasting 103

Introduction

The Keto Diet is the new trend in smart eating to lose weight – the reason why it has been able to capture such attention is because of its unique approach. The Keto Diet is all about eating high contents of fat and low contents of carb. When people first hear this they're always surprised because how can eating more fat make us slimmer? Well, that's because fats have been heavily stigmatized which is why all of us believe that it's only fats that make us fat when actually it's the carbs and sugars that we consume every day.

There are fats that are terrible for your body and you should avoid them, but there are also some good fats that help your body to absorb more vitamins and minerals from the food you consume. A high-fat diet doesn't just help you to lose weight, but also improves your cognitive abilities, cholesterol and even provides safety against many diseases.

The purpose of a keto is to make your eating habits a little more natural so that you stop consuming food that is artificial and fattening and instead consume food that is full of fats such as butter, cheese, nuts and fish.

In this book, you will learn everything about the keto diet – what it is all about, how it works, what are the benefits, how to follow it and how to keep yourself motivated.

Thanks again for purchasing this book, I hope you enjoy it!

Chapter One:
Ketogenic Diet Basics

Ketogenic diet is a diet that places and trains your body to be in a state wherein it primarily uses fat for energy. It achieves this through a natural metabolic process of your body called Ketosis that uses fat to create fuel for your body. A ketogenic diet has many similarities to the Atkins diet and many other low-carb diets. It has been known by several different names like low carb high fat, low carb diet and of course, the ketogenic diet.

The ketogenic diet can be implemented by discarding most of the sugars and starches in your diet and by eating healthy fats, moderate amounts of protein and very low carbs. With little carbohydrates in your diet, your body does not receive enough glucose to keep up with your body's caloric requirements. This eventually results in decreasing blood sugar levels in your body as it uses up glucose for its functions. When you eat foods that are high in carbs, your body automatically produces insulin and glucose. Insulin is made to process the glucose that is in your bloodstream by moving it around the body. Glucose is easy for your body to convert and be used for energy. Therefore, it gets chosen over all other energy sources.

As blood sugar level decreases, it looks for the stored glycogen present in your body and breaks it down to glucose and dissolves it in your blood to be distributed throughout your body. However, glycogen stores would also eventually run out. And when it does, your body would start to use fats as a source of energy for functions in its different parts and produce ketones when the liver processes it. Since glucose is used as the primary energy

3

source, the fat in your body isn't needed and gets stored. With a normal, high carb diet, your body uses glucose as its main form of energy. By lowering the carb intake, the body is put into ketosis. These fats could come from the food that you eat, from your meals or from the fat that your body stores. This is what is called ketosis.

When you hit ketosis, your body starts being very efficient at burning fat to create energy. It turns fat in the liver into ketones that supply energy to the brain. Many studies have shown that a keto diet can help you to improve your health and lose some weight. It can also help with Alzheimer's disease, epilepsy, cancer and diabetes.

The primary advantage of following a ketogenic diet is that it restores the capability of your body to use both fat and glucose as fuel to meet its energy or caloric needs. Your body is designed to use both glucose and fat as fuel. However, due to eating a high carbohydrate diet for most of their lives, many people lack the ability to use fat for the body's energy needs. This results in bodies that have a hard time maintaining a healthy weight and a healthy body fat percentage, both of which contribute to poor health. In fact, even if you are not overweight or obese, you may still have excess visceral fat, which is wrapped around your organs like your liver, pancreas and kidneys.

With a ketogenic diet, your body restores its flexibility to use both glucose and fat as fuel for its energy needs. This flexibility keeps your fat cells, both visceral and subcutaneous (the fat located under your skin and on top of your muscles), in check by using the stored energy found in those fat cells. This would, in turn, reduce the risks of having diseases involved with having high-fat stores, specifically visceral fat:

- Type 2 Diabetes
- Coronary Artery/ Heart Disease

- Colorectal Cancer
- Breast Cancer
- High Cholesterol
- High Blood Pressure
- Metabolic Syndrome
- Alzheimer's Disease
- Stroke
- Dementia

Other than decreasing risks of said diseases, this flexibility contributes to losing excess fat and weight in a manageable manner. Normally, while and after losing some weight, your body would feel less sated after eating the same meal you ate before the weight loss process started.

And in addition to this, you might feel an increase in appetite to compensate especially if you've been depriving yourself. However, when your body is in a state of ketosis, ketones help your body manage the hormones that decrease your satiety after meals and increase your appetite and hunger. With this, you lose weight without fighting your body to gain it back through its natural responses as to what it believes to be starvation.

Moreover, being able to utilize glucose and fat for energy prevents you from experiencing the big swings that affect your mental focus, making you hungry and irritable. When glucose runs out, ketones are readily available to fuel your brain. Even better, ketones give your brain a boost, enabling you to have better focus and concentration.

Lastly, the ketogenic diet has long been used for therapy of epilepsy. This diet has been recommended for children with uncontrolled epilepsy since the 1920's. It only disappeared from popular practice when the anti-seizure medication was made available. However, unlike the anti-seizure medicine currently available, the ketogenic diet does not cause extreme side effects on patients; like drowsiness, reduced concentration, personality changes and reduced brain function.

Starting Information & Tips

The Standard Ketogenic Diet (SKD) means that 70 percent of your diet should be in the form of healthy fats, 25 percent in the form of protein and 5 percent of carbohydrates. The percentages would be based on your daily caloric requirement that is unique for every person. Since you may need to increase your caloric intake due to higher needs, you may increase the percentage of healthy fats in your diet and your body can still achieve ketosis.

Other variations of the ketogenic diet that are tweaked based on certain needs are listed down below:

Targeted Ketogenic Diet (TKD)

This type of ketogenic diet is recommended for those who engage in physical fitness. In TKD, 30 to 60 minutes before exercise, you would eat the entirety of your carbohydrates for the day in one meal. The idea of this approach is to use the energy provided in this carbohydrate meal for your fitness activities before it disrupts your body's state of ketosis.

Cyclic Ketogenic Diet (CKD)

This approach is intended for people who have a high rate of physical activities like athletes and bodybuilders. When following CKD, you switch between a ketogenic diet, and after that you follow it with a few days of high carbohydrate consumption (9 to 12 times the carbohydrates in SKD), more commonly called, "carb loading." This approach takes advantage of the body's response to high blood sugar levels from a high carbohydrate diet, which is to store it in the body's muscles and fat cells. Having this abundance of stored energy and the body able to utilize both glucose and fat for energy, it can use this energy to keep the body going during high rates of physical activity.

High-Protein Ketogenic Diet

This is a method used to ease into a Standard Ketogenic Diet when the weight is beyond the normal levels. In this approach, your protein consumption in an SKD is increased by 10 percent and your fat consumption is reduced by 10 percent. This helps those with obesity to help suppress their appetite and reduce their food intake.

Restricted Ketogenic Diet:

This method was successfully used for a brain tumor patient. In this approach, carbohydrate and calorie intake are restricted for your body to deplete glycogen stores and to start producing ketones. Since cancer cells can only feed on glucose, they are starved to death while your body thrives on ketones. It starts with a water fasting regimen and proceeds to only have a Ketogenic Diet of 600 calories a day. After two months, ketosis is in full effect and no discernable brain tumor tissue can be detected.

Only the high protein ketogenic and the standard diets have had extensive studies done on them. The targeted and cyclical diets are more advanced and are only used by athletes and bodybuilders. Even though there are several different types of this diet, the standard ketogenic diet has been researched the most and is, therefore, the one that is usually recommended.

The reason why ketogenic diets are effective lies in the functional property of fat adaption. Your body needs to be told that it has to derive its energy from fats. The biggest challenge in this regard is to keep the body programmed to this state, on a regular basis. In order to maintain ketosis, here are a few tips that you must pay heed to.

Tip 1: Drink Enough Water

You must drink a healthy amount of water to maintain a healthy body. This is a fact that all of us know and are told about time and again. However, it has also proven to be the most difficult advice to follow. The modern lifestyle is so consuming that we mostly forget simple things like keeping our bodies hydrated and eating our meals on time. It is a good idea to drink around 4 glasses of water, first thing in the morning and another 4 glasses of water before the clock strikes noon.

Tip 2: Fast Once In A While

Like we said, our bodies fail to use up the fat stores because we never, ever fast. The body is pre-programmed to run ketosis as and when the body starves. Therefore, if you are finding it hard to get your body into ketosis or maintain the ketosis state of the body, you can fast intermittently. Fasting also helps in reducing food intake and manages appetites and cravings, both of which are crucial for your diet plan. However, be sure to go on a low-carb diet for a few days before fasting intermittently. The sudden lack of sugar in the body may land you up in a hypoglycemic state.

A daylong fast can be easily broken down into two phases. The first phase extends from the first meal you consume to the last meal you eat for the day. This is the build-up phase. The second phase, which extends from your last meal for the day to the first meal of the next day, is the cleansing phase. Ideally, the cleansing phase must be longer than the build-up phase. Whenever you fast, be sure to keep your body hydrated and eat good fats like butter and coconut oil. These additions play an instrumental role in boosting up the ketone production of the body and help to maintain a healthy insulin level.

Tip 3: Add Good Salts

The high insulin levels of the body, when it is in glycolysis, affect the functioning of the kidney in such a manner that the body retains sodium. As a result, the sodium-potassium ratio destabilizes. This is why most people are advised to reduce their sodium intake. On the other hand, when on a ketogenic diet, the insulin levels are normal and the kidney functioning allows sodium excretion more effectively.

As a result, the body needs sodium to ensure proper functioning. Never make the mistake of avoiding salts when running your body on a ketogenic diet. There are several ways by which you can increase the sodium levels of the body. Some of the best ways include having broth, eating sprouted pumpkin seeds, eating cucumber as part of the salad for natural sodium and adding a pinch of salt to almost everything you eat.

Tip 4: Exercise

Regular exercise can play a crucial role in maintaining the ketosis state of the body and avoiding deposition of glucose in body parts. Exercise allows activation of glucose transport molecules that facilitate deposition of glucose in the muscles and liver. Exercises like the ones used for resistance training also facilitate the maintenance of normal blood sugar levels.

It is important to understand in this context that overdoing exercise can result in the release of stress hormones. This, in turn, increases sugar levels of the body and destabilizes the ketosis state of the body. Regular and 'just-enough' exercise can be a great way to keep you on track.

Tip 5: Avoid Too Much Protein

Most regular diet programs recommend higher protein intake. However, excessive protein intake can initiate what is called gluconeogenesis, which again generates glucose. If you feel that your body is no longer able to maintain the ketosis state, you must take a keen look at the number of proteins that you are consuming. You may have more success with a much lower protein intake.

Tip 6: Choose What You Eat Wisely

Although the ketogenic diet recommends a reduced carbohydrate intake, it is not a good idea to remove carbs from the diet completely. Therefore, the inclusion of starchy vegetables and citric fruit is a good idea. On an odd day when you are off-ketosis, you can consume berries and potatoes. However, when on ketosis, be sure to avoid sweet potato and berry-type fruit completely.

Tip 7: Reduce Stress

Stress is the root cause of most of the problems that your body's face. In fact, an increase in the stress hormones in the body can pull you off ketosis because it increases the sugar levels substantially. Therefore, maintaining a ketosis state can be an uphill task if you are going through stressful times in your life. Managing stress is an important facet of the ketogenic diet. Adopt strategies that keep your stress levels in check if you wish to make your ketogenic diet work. In line with this objective, having adequate amounts of daily sleep and maintaining a stable lifestyle is also essential.

Who should follow this diet?

The keto diet is known in popular discourse only for weight loss, but it's about much more. In this section, we will look at who should follow this diet -

Epileptic Patients

The ketogenic diet was originally developed in the early 1900s as a means of controlling seizures in children. Fasting was long a treatment in treating epilepsy and doctors found that a high-fat diet helped mimic the metabolic response of fasting. They began treating epileptic children by feeding them a diet in which up to 90% of the calories came from fat and found a marked reduction in the seizures. Half of the children fed a ketogenic diet had a reduced number of seizures and about one in seven had a complete elimination of seizures altogether.

Some studies suggest that the ketones created by the ketogenic diet are the reason it is successful in treating epilepsy. Others believe that the depletion of glucose is the reason for its success. Whatever the reason, it has proven to be effective when medication has not.

The ketogenic diet, especially when used to treat seizures, is very intense and highly controlled and can be difficult for children to follow. Doctors usually only recommend it after multiple rounds of medication have proven unsuccessful. However, many of the epileptic children who are put on the ketogenic diet for two years or longer experience a reduction or elimination of seizures, even after they cease eating it. It does not seem to have the same effect in treating epileptic teenagers and adults, possibly because it is so strict and difficult to follow. However, they can still be treated with it as long as they are willing to follow it exactly.

The ketogenic diet for epilepsy is stricter than the ketogenic diet that many people are adhering to boost their health. Rather than a 70% fat this one requires 90% fats. Side effects can include stunted growth, constipation, kidney stones, weight loss and weaker bones. If the side effects become too much, a less intense but possibly less-effective diet, such as modified Atkins, can be implemented instead.

When an epileptic patient is starting out on the ketogenic diet, he or she may need to spend a few days in the hospital for monitoring to see what effects the diet is having. Close medical monitoring will be required, including keeping a food diary, corresponding with a dietitian and getting tested every one to three months. Hyper-vigilance for carbs is required, as they can show up in some very unexpected places. For example, most kinds of toothpaste and mouthwashes contain carbs.

Parents who place their epileptic children on a ketogenic diet will have to make substantial lifestyle changes. They will have to be able to implement the diet in such a way that the epileptic child does not see it as "unfair". He or she may see siblings enjoying sweets and feel left out. All caregivers, including babysitters, teachers and other family members, will have to be aware of the strict diet. Relatives who may want to "spoil" the child by giving him or her treats at family reunions will have to understand how serious the diet is, as one simple misstep or "cheat" can trigger seizures. Some creative ideas for handling these difficult situations include using treats other than food, such as toys, fun outings, or television time. Before Halloween one year, one dad of an epileptic child on the ketogenic diet sent out a letter to all of the homes in his neighborhood that explained why his son couldn't have candy and included a toy to give him instead. The heartwarming letter went viral.

When a medical professional advises getting off the ketogenic diet in favor of a more traditional diet that includes more carbs and protein, the transition will need to be made gradually. Especially in children, the body has become so adjusted to the ketogenic diet that the metabolic changes can be difficult to adapt to.

Type 1 Diabetics

Unlike Type 2 diabetes, Type 1 diabetes is actually an autoimmune disease in which the immune system attacks the pancreas and destroys the beta cells that detect blood sugar and create insulin. As a result, the body's cells are unable to absorb any glucose and blood sugar can build up to dangerously high levels. Type 1 diabetics usually must administer insulin through injections and constantly monitor their blood sugar levels to make sure they are within a safe range. While many people are diagnosed with it as children, half of those diagnosed are over the age of 30.

There are many complications that people with Type 1 diabetes can experience, possibly as a result of the autoimmune dysfunction rather than insulin deficiency. High blood pressure and blood sugar levels can lead to eye damage, such as diabetic retinopathy, nerve damage, kidney damage and heart disease. The challenge in successfully responding to Type 1 diabetes is not only regulating blood sugar and insulin levels but also dealing with the autoimmune problems that can lead to further complications.

Lifestyle is the most important factor in managing Type 1 diabetes. Avoiding sugar, getting regular exercise, being
consistent with insulin injections and being aware of the symptoms of impending problems are some of the most crucial things. Lowering blood sugar, thereby lowering the need for insulin, can be very effective at managing the disease.
The ketogenic diet can be a powerful way of lowering blood sugar in patients with Type 1 diabetes. Many find that they are able to reduce their need for insulin by up to 80% or more.

When following a ketogenic diet with Type 1 diabetes, the person must be absolutely all in. There are no cheats allowed, as just one cheat meal can put the body in a dangerous, potentially deadly state known as ketoacidosis. This occurs when ketones build up in the blood, causing it to become more acidic.

The ketones, which are naturally present on the ketogenic diet, can build up to dangerously high levels as they react with the blood sugar. Diabetics on the ketogenic diet should closely monitor their ketone and glucose levels and remain carefully under a doctor's supervision.

Type 1 diabetics may need to follow a modified version of the ketogenic diet, which is more strictly controlled but more suited to the disease.

Type 2 Diabetics

Type 2 diabetes, also known as adult diabetes, is oftentimes the result of lifestyle choices that lead to chronically high levels of blood sugar, thereby leading to insulin resistance. While Type 1 diabetes is caused by the inability of the body to create insulin, Type 2 diabetes is the result of it being unable to use insulin. Increasingly unhealthy lifestyle choices are leading to children being diagnosed with Type 2 diabetes, whereby it was previously unheard of in people under the age of 50.

Diet, exercise and close monitoring of insulin levels are key to managing Type 2 diabetes. Complete lifestyle overhauls have led some people to completely reverse the symptoms and no longer need medication. The most obvious benefit is that the lowered blood sugar leads to less dependence on insulin.

The conundrum created by applying the ketogenic diet to Type 2 diabetes is that because so many people with the disease are overweight or obese, adopting a high-fat diet seems to be counterintuitive. After all, fat is a much more concentrated source of calories than carbs or protein, so it should actually lead to weight gain and exacerbate the person's health problems. However, that is a myth based on a misunderstanding of calories and the complex chemistry involved in metabolism. The fact is that not all calories are created equal and healthy fats, as opposed to carbs, can actually decrease your appetite so that you end up consuming fewer calories. Additionally, the decreased production of ghrelin, the hunger hormone and the increased production of leptin and amylin, the satiety hormones, generated by the state of ketosis further restrict the calorie intake.

As with Type 1 diabetes, people with Type 2 diabetes are at risk of developing ketoacidosis, so constant monitoring of blood sugar and ketones is important. Additionally, the ketogenic diet should be followed under a doctor's supervision.

Early-Stage Alzheimer's Patients

One of the biggest health concerns today is the risk of developing Alzheimer's disease. Alzheimer's seems to have a bit of a genetic component and is also linked with lifestyle factors. As previously mentioned, some researchers have come to call it Type 3 Diabetes because of its connection with insulin resistance and a buildup of glucose in the brain.

Preliminary studies, both in animal and human trials, indicate that the ketogenic diet is effective at restoring normal brain metabolism in people with early-stage Alzheimer's disease. It reduces and can even eliminate the buildup of unabsorbed glucose that leads to cell death while providing the brain with the superior energy provided by ketones. Ketones are able to provide all of the nutrients necessary for optimal brain function. At optimal levels they do not build up in the bloodstream, leading to the creation of the dangerous plaques and tangles that cause neurodegeneration.

As yet, there is no indication that the ketogenic diet can reverse Alzheimer's disease once it has begun. However, results so far are promising. Research over the past few decades has revealed that the brain has a high level of plasticity, meaning that neurons are able to regenerate, grow and adapt to changing needs. Ketones may be able to tap into this plasticity to help halt Alzheimer's in its tracks and future research into treatment for Alzheimer's will focus heavily on ketones.

People who are diagnosed with Alzheimer's disease tend to be older, usually over the age of 60, so implementing the changes required by the ketogenic diet can be difficult. Additionally, maintaining the person's lifestyle as much as possible is seen as a cornerstone in caring for someone with Alzheimer's, as consistency and normalcy can help deal with the emotional challenges that people with the disease face. Getting Alzheimer's patients to establish a ketogenic diet can be very difficult and will require the complete commitment of all caregivers.

People, who are at risk of developing Alzheimer's disease, because of preexisting insulin resistance, genetic factors, or environmental factors, may benefit from the ketogenic diet. It may prevent the brain decay that is characteristic of the disease.

Parkinson's Patients

Parkinson's disease is a neurodegenerative disorder caused by abnormal levels of the hormone dopamine. The dopamine-creating neurons die and the loss of dopamine results in the characteristic tremors that people with

Parkinson's experience. Additionally, they deal with problems such as depression, lack of clarity, forgetfulness and loss of physical function. The disease is progressive, so it gets worse over time. Medications are available to help manage the symptoms, but there is no cure.

Dysfunction in the mitochondria is believed to be a cause of the death of the dopamine-creating neurons, which leads to Parkinson's. The previous chapter already discussed the role of ketones in protecting and enhancing the mitochondria, so from this perspective, ketones may play a role in helping to treat Parkinson's patients. Preliminary studies in animals have shown that the ketogenic diet can improve mitochondrial function. In humans, a preliminary study has shown that one month on the ketogenic diet leads to decreased tremors, elevated mood, improved gait and increased energy.

People who are diagnosed with Parkinson's disease tend to be older, so implementing the intense lifestyle changes required by the ketogenic diet can be quite difficult. Those who participated in the preliminary testing had trouble staying on it and several quit, despite the potential for treatment. A gradual transition to the ketogenic diet may be helpful in maintaining it.

Cancer Patients

In addition to finding new medications that can potentially help cancer patients, much cancer research is now looking into the effects of diet and lifestyle as supplements to traditional treatments. Vegetable juicing and eating an organic-only diet has helped many cancer patients recover. New research is focusing on the potential of a ketogenic diet in helping to cure cancer.

One way that a ketogenic diet may benefit cancer patients is that sugar is all but eliminated. Sugar is basically what cancer cells thrive on; there is a direct correlation between sugar consumption and growth of tumors. By switching the body's energy source from glucose to ketones, the tumors become starved and may shrink.

Additionally, the benefits for mitochondrial metabolism may improve the responses of healthy cells and generate apoptosis, the body's method of intentionally destroying cancerous cells. Studies are showing that a ketogenic diet increases the oxidative stress on the mitochondria in cancer cells, making them more sensitive to chemotherapy and other traditional treatments.

Meanwhile, the mitochondria of the healthy cells are enhanced, making them less prone to the harmful effects of treatments. Cancer patients who want to adopt a ketogenic diet should consult with an oncologist who specializes in how a ketogenic diet can help with that particular type of cancer.

PCOS Patients

Polycystic ovarian syndrome, or PCOS, is a metabolic dysfunction that is closely correlated with insulin resistance. It leads to problems such as infertility, acne, dysmenorrhea (heavy periods that have intense cramping), amenorrhea (lack of periods) and hirsutism (irregular hair growth across the body). While the ovaries usually release an egg every 28 days, in women with PCOS, the eggs remain in the ovaries and turn into cysts. Over time, the cysts build up in both ovaries until there are dozens or even hundreds. Many women with PCOS treat their symptoms with medication, but the disease can also be managed and sometimes even reversed through diet.

Consistently high levels of blood sugar cause insulin resistance. The first step to treating PCOS through diet is by eliminating sugar, then reducing and eliminating all other carbs, as well. PCOS is also strongly correlated with obesity; some women develop PCOS and become obese because of the intense hormonal disruptions, while some obese women are more prone to developing PCOS. Another step towards treating the disease with diet is to lose weight. Because the weight gain tends to be at least partly hormonal, balancing the hormones is crucial.

The ketogenic diet can help women with PCOS to both balance their hormones and lose weight. Although clinical studies are few and small, case studies and anecdotal evidence regarding the success of low-carb diets in treating PCOS are impressive; the lowered insulin levels help to reverse insulin resistance and stabilize other hormone imbalances. It is not uncommon for women with PCOS who are on a low-carb diet to lose weight, achieve normal periods and even regain their fertility.

While there is little research as to the ketogenic diet specifically with women who have PCOS, preliminary results are promising. There are several foods on the ketogenic diet, such as fatty fish and nuts that are particularly helpful for those with the disease. If you have PCOS and want to try the ketogenic diet to see if it can help relieve your symptoms and even reverse the disease, talk with your endocrinologist about how it may benefit you.

People with Autism

Autism is a neurological disorder that has been on the rise, particularly in the United States. Its characteristic feature is impaired social interaction and cognitive development, including language development. The increased prevalence of autistic diagnoses has led many parents to be concerned about possible causes of autism. Some have even shunned life-saving vaccines because they are concerned that they may cause autism. Its causes seem to be varied and include genetic and environmental factors.

Treatment usually focuses on managing behavior with intense therapy; there is no known cure for autism. It is a lifelong condition and many adults with autism must either be cared for full time by a family member or live in a care home. The success of the ketogenic diet in treating neurological disorders has led to speculation about whether it may be able to benefit people with autism. Many diets have been applied to clinical studies for children with autism spectrum disorders, but the benefits seem to be minimal. However, the ketogenic diet seems to hold great promise and has already proven to help autistic children in some clinical trials.

It is not uncommon for people with autism to also suffer from seizures. The benefits of the ketogenic diet in treating seizures were described in the first section; someone with autism who also has seizures may experience diminished epileptic activity as a result of the ketogenic diet.

Autism spectrum disorders tend to display certain behaviors, including repetitive behaviors known as stimming and agitation. Mice with characteristics that mimic autism, such as repetitive behaviors and lack of social interaction, who were fed a ketogenic diet experienced reversals of the symptoms and behaved like normal mice. In clinical trials, autistic children fed a ketogenic diet experienced marked improvement in these behaviors and even showed an increase in social activity.

Autism also tends to have an effect on cognition. While some forms of autism, such as Asperger's syndrome, can lead to increased mental acuity, there is oftentimes a lack of executive function, which inhibits the person's ability to make connections between ideas. The ketogenic diet has been shown to help people with autism improve their cognitive process. This may be because it promotes the neurotransmitter adenosine, which promotes sleep and reduces anxious behavior.

People with Mood Disorders and Mental Illness

The typical Western diet, which is high in processed foods, sugars and other carbs, triggers biological processes that induce mood disorders like depression and anxiety. Sugar is possibly the most addictive substance on the planet, so it is little wonder that it would cause problems with mood. Many people rely on antidepressants and other medications to deal with their mood disorders; however, they can also be treated naturally. Eliminating sugar is the first step. Following a ketogenic diet can dramatically improve mood.

Additionally, the neurological processes stimulated by a ketogenic diet can treat more severe mental illnesses, such as bipolar and schizophrenia. While going keto is unlikely to cure the disease, it can help to manage symptoms.

It is important to remember that mood disorders and mental illnesses are multifaceted and can be triggered by stressful events and other environmental factors; they also seem to have a genetic link. While improving the brain's chemistry, a ketogenic diet is unable to resolve these other factors that contribute to mental illness and mood disorders.

Depression:
As opposed to sadness, which is a normal emotion that everyone experiences; depression is a clinical condition in which a lowered mood persists for weeks, months and even years. It results in a severely lowered quality of life both for the depressed individual and his or her family.

Numerous case studies exist to support the idea that a ketogenic diet can help treat depression and these case studies seem to be backed by scientific evidence and data. One cause of depression is neurotoxicity spurred by imbalances of the neurotransmitters GABA and glutamate. The use of ketones is able to improve the balance, thereby alleviating some of the chemical causes of depression.

Additionally, depression and inflammation are strongly linked. Conditions such as leaky gut syndrome, which is becoming more prevalent among Westerners eating a high-carb diet, decimate the microbiome of the gut, which is responsible for much of the hormones that the body produces. This alone can lead to the chemical imbalances that are associated with depression. Leaky gut syndrome and a less-than-optimal microbiome also contribute to inflammation, which can also cause or worsen depression. The ketogenic diet eliminates the foods that lead to intestinal problems, making it ideal to treat some of the causes of depression.

Adapting a ketogenic diet is just one aspect of overcoming depression and it is not a substitute for counseling.

Anxiety:

While some stress is beneficial and necessary for daily function, anxiety refers to a large amount of stress that hampers a person to complete the tasks he or she needs to do and lowers the overall quality of life. The build-up of stress hormones, such as cortisol and adrenaline, can cause stressful events to affect a person's metabolic processes. In addition to depression, anxiety-related disorders are on the rise, especially in children, who are constantly expected to achieve increasingly high expectations. The high-sugar diet adopted by many Westerners is known to contribute to anxiety and also fuels the release of cortisol and adrenaline. Eliminating sugar and exercising regularly are important to reducing levels of stress hormones. The ketogenic diet can also help stabilize the metabolic processes that lead to anxiety and reverse the damage caused by it.

As with depression, there are numerous case studies of people who suffered from anxiety and experienced substantial relief from following a ketogenic diet. This is possible because the metabolic processes in the brain are transformed through the creation and burning of ketones for energy instead of using sugar.

Schizophrenia:

Schizophrenia is a rare but serious mental illness in which a person experiences things that are not present as if they are happening. They typically experience hallucinations, which are not limited to seeing things that are not present but can also include hearing things (the "voices" associated with schizophrenia) and feeling sensations, such as itching, that do not have a physical cause. The exact causes are not known, but there seem to be both genetic and environmental factors. Treatment for schizophrenia includes behavior modification therapy and heavy medication regimens.

People suffering from schizophrenia are at a high risk of suicide and also of harming others; many need full-time care throughout their entire lives. In laboratory trials, mice whose brains were induced to have the same chemical structure as a schizophrenic brain and who had schizophrenic behaviors were fed a ketogenic diet. After three weeks, some of their mental processes became completely normal. While there is presently no data to support the treatment of schizophrenic humans with a ketogenic diet, there is certainly promise.

Bipolar:

Bipolar is a serious mental illness in which a person swings from periods of depression to mania. Intense manic periods can cause the person to become completely detached from reality and engage in risky behaviors that he or she would not ordinarily consider. There is a high rate of suicide and other harmful behaviors associated with bipolar disorder and while some people with bipolar are able to function on their own, others need lifelong care.

Many bipolar medications are also used to treat epilepsy. Because of the ketogenic diet's success in treating epilepsy, researchers were interested to find if it could also treat bipolar. Scientific evidence says that yes, it may be able to. Seizure medications that reduce the amount of sodium in the extracellular area are the only ones that are effective at treating bipolar; the ketogenic diet is effective at achieving the same thing.

Sodium is responsible for many of the metabolic processes that occur within the brain, as keeping an optimal balance of sodium and potassium is necessary for ensuring the correct electrical function that enables communication between neurons. Whacked-out sodium levels can cause problems with the functioning of neurons, which can trigger the psychotic episodes associated with bipolar. This is the reason why bipolar medication seeks to stabilize the brain's sodium.

By helping the brain maintain optimal sodium levels, both within neurons and outside of them, the ketogenic diet is able to achieve the same effect as bipolar medication.

People with Cerebral Palsy

Cerebral palsy is a neurological condition that is usually caused by lack of oxygen during birth or during the first five years of life. The brain damage caused by the lack of oxygen can lead to problems including seizures, lack of coordination, muscle spasms, difficulty with depth perception, speech difficulties and hearing and vision problems. There is no cure for cerebral palsy, but a ketogenic diet can be part of a treatment plan to improve the quality of life for people who have it.

The ketogenic can be hugely effective at treating the seizures that are associated with cerebral palsy. Further research into how it can help other aspects of cerebral palsy, such as brain damage and muscle spasms, is necessary to see how effective it is as a global treatment.

People Who Want To Lose Weight

The body's chemistry, not the arithmetic of calories in versus calories out, is what determines whether people gain weight or lose weight. Consuming carbs leads to the production of insulin, which turns on the body's fat-producing hormones. Research is increasingly finding that insulin is directly related to weight gain. Unless you immediately burn off the sugars that you consume, they will be stored as fat. This occurs regardless of whether you are eating "diet" foods or not. The key to losing weight is not in restricting calories but in lowering your insulin levels.

People on the ketogenic diet often find that they lose weight without having to restrict calories. They feel less hungry, have a much more stable appetite and feel more satisfied after eating. Without sugar being used as the body's primary fuel source, they immediately begin to burn through fat.

Some doctors have suggested that people on the ketogenic diet immediately begin to lose water weight rather than actual fat. However, this claim comes back to the faulty reasoning about the body needing carbs for energy in the form of glucose. The ketogenic diet leads the body to respond as if it is in a state of fasting by burning through fat at a high rate.

People with Fatty Liver Disease

The liver is an organ that is part of the digestive system; it filters out toxins, synthesizes enzymes and other chemicals necessary for digestion, breaks down carbs and even helps with blood clotting! It is a very important organ and keeping it healthy is of the utmost importance. Fatty liver disease is the first in a progression of liver problems. One type is caused by alcohol consumption and the other type is correlated with genetics, obesity, cholesterol and consumption of carbohydrates. Symptoms include fatigue, weight loss, nausea, confusion, lack of clarity and overall weakness. Left untreated, it could turn into cirrhosis or scarring of the liver. Cirrhosis is a serious disease that causes fluids to accumulate throughout the body, muscles to atrophy, internal bleeding, liver failure and jaundice.

While alcohol-based fatty liver disease is treated by completely abstaining from alcohol, non-alcoholic fatty liver disease (NAFLD) can be treated through diet. Adopting a high-fat diet seems to be counter-intuitive for treating a disease characterized by the fat build-up in the liver; carbs are actually more often the culprit behind NAFLD. People with NAFLD who adopt the ketogenic diet have shown reductions in the fats in their livers and overall better liver function.

If you have NAFLD and want to get on the ketogenic diet, make sure you inform your doctor. He or she may recommend frequent testing to monitor how the diet is affecting your liver.

People with Acne

Acne is a skin condition that results from unbalanced hormones, especially insulin and cortisol. Insulin causes the creation of new skin cells and causes them to stick together, both of which can lead to breakouts. It also stimulates the production of sebum, which is a type of oil the skin produces and testosterone, which also causes acne.

Severely reducing insulin levels by following a ketogenic diet has been shown to drastically help people who suffer from acne. The thought of following a high-fat diet to decrease the skin's oil production seems counterintuitive, but again, it all comes back to the body's complex chemistry and metabolism.

Many people find that when they first begin the ketogenic diet, their acne actually gets worse. However, this is usually because hormone levels are stabilizing and inflammation is healing. A month or so in, acne begins to heal and, with time, even the scars begin to go away.

People with ADD, ADHD and Executive Dysfunctions

ADD, or attention deficit disorder and ADHD, attention deficit and hyperactive disorder, cause many children and adults to have difficulty focusing and staying on task. While some people think of the disorders as people just not being willing to sit still and be quiet, they are actually rooted in neurological processes that involve neurotransmitters and other aspects of the brain's chemistry. They are often treated with medication, although some people prefer to treat them through lifestyle and forego medication. Executive function disorders are common in people with ADD and ADHD. Think of all of the functions that an executive at an office must perform: delegate tasks to employees, manage a busy schedule, coordinate meetings, oversee various departments, etc. Imagine an office trying to function without an executive and all of the different parts are running but not being coordinated. That is what an executive function disorder looks like. People with an executive function disorder know what they need to do, but they are unable to figure out exactly how to carry out the tasks.

The ketogenic diet can be of benefit to people struggling with these disorders. Parents of children with these disorders usually restrict sugar intake, as it can lead to an increase in symptoms. Consumption of whole foods without any preservatives can help decrease symptoms, as can eating high levels of healthy fats. While there haven't been many clinical trials done regarding the benefits of the ketogenic diet for ADD, ADHD and executive function disorders, there are numerous case studies suggesting that it can be very helpful.

People with a History of Eating Disorders

Eating disorders are not primarily physical but rather psychiatric problems. They tend to have deep roots in self-image, self-esteem, self-confidence and social wellbeing. The most common eating disorder is anorexia, a condition in which sufferers have an irrational fear of weight gain and see themselves as much larger than they actually are. They starve themselves and as a result, have severe nutrient deficiencies and are severely underweight. Left untreated, anorexics can die from the disorder. People with anorexia typically have an intense fear of fat, even though carbs are much more of a culprit in terms of weight gain. Because they are in a state of starvation (as opposed to fasting), they crave sweets and may binge eat on fat-free carbs. Eating a high-fat diet is not a good idea for someone who has been struggling with anorexia.

Additionally, because it promotes weight loss, anorexics should avoid it. Another common eating disorder is bulimia, a condition in which someone binge eats and then induces either vomiting or diarrhea to rid the body of all of the calories consumed. The severe instability that the body faces can make the ketogenic diet quite dangerous. However, if done under the careful supervision of a physician and psychiatrist, people with bulimia can find that the ketogenic diet is actually very healing for both their minds and their bodies. This must be done as part of a comprehensive treatment program and not a method of losing weight (as a substitute for purging).

People with Gallbladder Problems

People with gallbladder problems or with no gallbladder should avoid the ketogenic diet because they have difficulty processing fats. The gallbladder stores bile, a chemical that helps break down fats in the intestines. With the decreased levels of bile, the fat is unable to be absorbed and a nutrient deficiency results. Additionally, the ketogenic diet can lead to gallstones, which can exacerbate existing gallbladder problems.

However, under a doctor's careful supervision, people with gallbladder issues can take some steps to enable them to follow the ketogenic diet successfully. Consuming foods that stimulate the production of bile and optimal levels of stomach acid, such as ginger, celery, cucumbers, apple cider vinegar, artichokes, asparagus and dandelion greens can help avoid some of the problems with fat absorption. Drinking plenty of water — four cups within the first hour of waking up and an additional four cups before lunch — is essential. This will mean a lot of trips to the bathroom, so you will have to decide if your lifestyle will allow you to follow the ketogenic diet with gallbladder issues.

People Who Have Had Bariatric Surgery

After having stomach-altering surgery, such as a gastric bypass, the ketogenic diet can prove to be challenging. People who have had bariatric surgery have usually struggled with morbid obesity for much of their lives and have spent just as much time trying out different diets in the attempt to lose weight. The problem is that when they are successful at losing weight, they are equally successful at gaining it back.

While the ketogenic diet provides the benefit of weight loss, it is not primarily a weight-loss tool. When people who have been on the ketogenic diet revert back to eating a moderate amount of carbs, they tend to gain back some of the weight that they lose. For someone who has had bariatric surgery, this means getting back onto the weight-loss, weight-gain roller coaster. The results can be demoralizing, especially after so much effort was put into the weight-loss surgery.

Instead, people who have had bariatric surgery are usually advised to follow a modified ketogenic diet, which allows for a high protein intake rather than a high fat intake. If you have had bariatric surgery, consult with your physician about how you can get your body into a state of ketosis without getting back onto the weight-loss, weight-gain roller coaster.

People with Kidney Problems

While the ketogenic diet is unlikely to cause harmful effects for people who don't have kidney problems, those who have pre-existing issues are more likely to experience complications. Your kidneys are the organs that filter your blood and remove toxins and other waste products to be excreted as urine. You only need one functioning kidney to live, but people who have a history of kidney problems tend to have an issue with both.

Diets that are high in protein tend to be harder on the kidneys because they cause them to work more to excrete the excess calcium, potassium, sodium and by-products of metabolizing proteins. The process of ketosis can cause kidney stones to form and also causes the blood to become more acidic, leading to potential complications for those with a kidney condition. Left untreated, kidney problems can lead to a need for dialysis, a time-consuming and taxing procedure in which the blood is artificially filtered a few times each week.

If you have pre-existing kidney problems but want to follow the ketogenic diet, consult with your doctor and only change your diet under his or her supervision. You may need to be monitored and tested frequently to ensure that the diet is not harming your kidneys.

People Who Are Underweight

While obesity is the primary factor behind many chronic diseases and is reaching epidemic proportions, there are many people who are actually underweight. This may be because of metabolic problems, such as hyperthyroidism, an intense exercise regimen, or not consuming enough calories to meet the body's nutritional needs. There could also be serious underlying health problems, especially if a person with a normal weight begins to lose weight without making any lifestyle changes. Unexpected weight loss can signal serious problems, including diabetes and cancer.

The ketogenic diet is known to induce weight loss, so even though it is much healthier than many other diets, it can have a negative effect on people who are already underweight. If you are underweight and want to begin the ketogenic diet for its health benefits, speak with your doctor. He or she may advise that you adopt a modified ketogenic diet, which will include more carbs and protein to help you gain weight while eating more foods that will induce ketosis.

People Who Should Avoid the Ketogenic Diet

If you are under any medication, breastfeeding, or have any degenerative disease, please see a doctor who understands the ketogenic diet. Your health could be aggravated due to your condition. The ketogenic diet is for the purposes of improving your health and not making things worse. It's better to be safe and consult your doctor than be sorry about it just because you failed to have a consultation.

Chapter Two:
Understanding the Keto Diet

To understand how the keto diet works, you must first know how your body converts the food that you eat into energy and how it uses it. This is done by your digestive system through digestion. Digestion is the process of breaking down food through mechanical and chemical actions. Without breaking down food into their simpler forms, your body cannot use it for energy, growth and cell repair. The food that you eat consists of nutrients that can be primarily divided into two classifications: macronutrients and micronutrients. While micronutrients help our body to repair, grow and protect itself, macronutrients provide the energy our body needs. These two nutrient subdivisions could be further divided - the macronutrients into fats, proteins and carbohydrates; and micronutrients into the vast array of vitamins and minerals.

Carbohydrates

Carbohydrates come from sugars, starches and fiber found in the fruit, grains and vegetables that you eat. These are broken down by the saliva in your mouth, small intestine and pancreas into glucose, sucrose and fructose (simple sugars). The simple sugars are for the body's immediate energy needs.

Protein

Proteins come from meat, eggs and beans that you eat. These are all broken down by the stomach, small intestines and pancreas into amino acids.

These are used by your body to create neurotransmitters, non-essential amino acids and other protein-based compounds. Excess amino acids are circulated and used to repair damaged tissues or are stored as glucose.

Fats

Fats come from oils and fat in our diet. These are broken down by the liver and pancreas into fatty acids and glycerol. These are used by the body to repair cells and make different chemicals or tissues.

Vitamins

Vitamins come from the food solids and liquid that you eat. As these are broken down by your system, the small and large intestines absorb the vitamins for use in different body functions, from fighting inflammation to repairing cell damage. These are all absorbed in the small intestines by specialized cells that pass across the intestinal lining. Your bloodstream circulates amino acids, simple sugars, glycerol and other salts and vitamins to your liver. The vessels that move white blood cells and lymph throughout the body, called as lymphatic system, circulates fatty acids and vitamins.

This whole process of digestion is controlled by your nervous system and the hormones your body produce. Your nerves cause muscles of the GI tract to contract or relax to digest food and release a substance to control the movement of food and the production of digestive juices. Your hormones, on the other hand, regulate appetite and stimulate the production of digestive juices.

There will be excess nutrients that your body won't need after this whole ordeal. Your excess blood sugar and amino acids would be stored in your body as either glycogen in liver, muscle and fat cells. The excess amino acids get stored as glucose while the excess fats get stored as triglycerides in the fat cells. Vitamins in excess are either expelled through urine, if water-soluble, or stored in the liver and fat cells, if fat-soluble.

The Fasted State

Around 2 to 8 hours after your last meal, your body enters a state of fasting. In this state, your body's blood sugar drops to a lower threshold level, which also brings down the levels of insulin in it. With the drop of glucose in your blood, a hormone from the liver, called glucagon is released to release the stored energy in your cells. This raises your glucose levels in your bloodstream, which is primarily used by the brain and red blood cells.

After these stores are used up, the body starts to be in a state of ketosis. Triglycerides are released from fat cells and are used by your muscles and liver cells as fuel. From the liver's use of triglycerides, ketones are formed and used if more energy is needed. As your body's fasted state goes further, more triglycerides are released, broken down and used for energy. As you can see, thanks to ketosis, the body can freely switch energy consumption from blood sugar to the stored glycogen, glucose and triglycerides. However, due to the high carbohydrate diets, your body had somehow gotten used to only using blood sugar for energy.

Whenever it goes down, you start getting hungry and craving for a meal with carbohydrates. If you do eat a meal without carbohydrates, you don't feel as satisfied. This does not normally occur when ketosis occurs in a fasted state due to the ketones that prevent hunger hormones from coming out and trigger hormones that signal your brain to feel sated as if you ate a meal.

Ketosis Effect

On a diet that is high or centered around carbohydrates, your body is primarily burning glucose for fuel. Since it is frequently supplied with carbohydrates through your meals, it does not adapt itself out of a glucose burning state and into fat burning. And whenever it needs more glucose, your body would just tell you that it's time to eat. As any excess in caloric intake would result in your body storing fat, it would just keep storing fat whenever you do. Since it is in a standard state of using glucose as a primary source of energy, your body won't readily use what is in its fat stores. This perpetuates a cycle of your body gaining fat from the excess caloric intake and being unable to burn it for energy.

With a ketogenic diet, the body does not primarily depend on carbohydrates for your body's daily caloric requirements. This results in your body adapting to this diet and, then naturally, switching to looking for its required energy and primarily using fat for fuel. With your body in a state of ketosis, it uses up your fat stores more readily whenever your body runs out of the fat it got from your last meal. Instead of you feeling hungry, it just uses up the stored energy in your body fat.

There are two ways that you can do for your body to achieve a state of ketosis. This is through fasting from food or substituting the carbohydrates in your diet with healthy fats, which is what the ketogenic diet does. Since fasting in the long-term is not a sustainable way to achieve ketosis, the ketogenic diet is the way to go for anyone who wants to take advantage of this fat burning state of your body. However, the ketogenic diet goes beyond the ratio of the carbohydrates, proteins and fats that are in your meals. You must eat the right nutrients to be able to healthily achieve ketosis. Doing so otherwise could lead to chronic inflammation, metabolic disorders and other degenerative diseases.

Chapter Three:
Benefits of Keto Diet

The ketogenic diet is absolutely unique and it gives you benefits that you wouldn't find in any other diet. The main aim behind the diet is to reduce your dependence on carbohydrates and inducing your body to burn more fats.

Fighting Cancer

The ketogenic diet is a natural deterrent for cancer cells. The ketogenic diet usually consists of 75 percent fat, 20 percent protein and 5 percent carbohydrates. This limits the number of carbs and sugar that you consume. Cancer cells replicate themselves throughout your body once they start growing. These cells need sugar in order to create enough energy to replicate themselves. Since the ketogenic diet eliminates intake of sugar, the cancer cells are left stranded.

The diet also reduces your intake of carbohydrates. This further helps in fighting cancer, as the cancer cells do not have an alternative source to generate energy. This does not mean that you won't have the energy that you need for daily activities. Your regular cells can use fats to generate energy but cancer cells cannot simply switch to a different source.

Helps in Weight Loss

If we consume carbohydrates, insulin is released throughout the body in order to increase blood glucose. Insulin is a type of hormone. Its basic function is to ensure that the body has enough energy for all of its needs. So, when insulin is released it further propagates the cells to save as much energy as possible. The cells initially save the energy in the form of glycogen (carbohydrates in their stored form) then later on as fat.

The ketogenic diet aims at reducing the level of carbohydrates that you consume so that they are almost negligible in your body. This prevents your body from releasing insulin. When insulin is not released in the body then there is a lack of glycogen, which the body needs in order to generate energy. Your body is forced to burn fats in order to generate energy. This helps in reducing the number of fats that are stored in your body and therefore, helps you to lose weight.

Treating Alzheimer's disease

Alzheimer is a disease that slowly deteriorates your nervous system. If it goes untreated it can even lead to Dementia. The ketogenic diet is the perfect way to treat Alzheimer's.

When you get old, the nervous system stops working properly and tends to slow down after a while. This causes mood swings, random episodes of dementia and most importantly memory loss. To prevent Alzheimer's from growing, it's important to take care of your nervous system.

The nervous system is directly linked to the brain. So, to help the brain it is important to consume healthy fats. Healthy fats make your brain more active. The ketogenic diet consists of 70 percent healthy fats and therefore it helps the brain.

Lower Blood Pressure

Elevated blood pressure can lead to many diseases including heart attack, kidney failure and others.

The ketogenic diet makes sure that you do not consume too many carbs. This reduces the blood pressure of your body. It's been seen in numerous cases that a reduction in consumption of carbs led to decreased blood pressure. The reason behind this is that a low carb diet induces the body to store fewer fluids. This includes the constituent fluids present in the blood.

A lower blood pressure reduces the risk of an early death and also makes you feel more energetic than before.

Improved brain function

The idea that the brain functions entirely on glucose is simply untrue. The brain only needs about 40 grams of glucose per day (that level may vary according to the individual), which can be synthesized from proteins through the process of gluconeogenesis. Once the body becomes fully adapted to the ketogenic diet, the brain can meet 75% of its energy needs from ketones, with the remaining 25% coming from the glucose made from proteins.

The brain actually contains astrocytes, which produce ketones. This fact indicates that the brain actually does function more optimally on ketones. Also, the fact that the ketogenic diet was originally established to treat neurological disorders, especially epilepsy, shows how important they are to establishing optimal brain function.

Ketones are actually a more efficient fuel for the brain and create fewer waste products than glucose.

Over time, the brain clears out all of the waste products generated by relying on glucose for energy. Running on ketones, it is able to establish optimal sodium levels between neurons, thereby decreasing the symptoms of diseases like depression, anxiety, schizophrenia and bipolar. Damaged neurons can begin to heal and even regenerate. Thoughts become clearer, mood increases and the brain operates optimally.

Improved nutrition

Without eating many fruit and limiting the vegetables consumed, one concern about the ketogenic diet is that over time, it can lead to nutrient deficiencies. While it may be beneficial in the short term to help achieve weight loss and other health goals, over the long term, it can be harmful because it does not provide complete nutrition. The only thing necessary to induce ketosis is very few carbs and lots of fat. This can be accomplished by drinking canola oil (which is not natural at all, as there is no such thing as a canola plant), eating margarine (which is made from trans fats) and pushing down hot dogs. Eating like this will certainly create severe nutrient deficiencies and cause illness.

However, a proper approach to the ketogenic diet, which includes lots of fatty cuts from high-quality meat produced from animals that are raised organically, nuts, leafy green vegetables, dairy, butter, olive oil and avocados, the diet is actually very nutrient dense. In fact, you will be consuming much more vitamins and minerals than in a typical American diet.

Lower cholesterol and risk of heart disease

The scary fact behind heart disease is that it is caused by eating carbs, not fats. Increasing research is revealing that heart disease rates are higher in people who eat a lot of carbs, even though traditional advice is that people with risk factors for heart disease should limit their fat intake. Carbs raise blood triglycerides, the dangerous fats that float through your bloodstream and can cause blockages when they build up to dangerous levels. Additionally, growing evidence suggests that carbs, not fats, raise the bad LDL cholesterol that can also clog arteries. The more carbs you eat, the higher your risk of heart disease.

There is a lot of misunderstanding about how cholesterol actually works. It is necessary for bodily function and is produced naturally; the body's cholesterol levels are actually affected very little by the foods that we eat. The carriers of the cholesterol are either the high-density lipoproteins (HDL) or low-density lipoproteins (LDL), which are determined by the foods that we eat. Eating a lot of cholesterol doesn't increase chances of heart disease.

Triglycerides are the fats that are stored in your fat cells but can also accumulate in the bloodstream. They can also accumulate in the liver, leading to fatty liver disease. They are produced from glucose, so the best way to lower your triglycerides is to severely restrict the carbs that you are consuming. Numerous studies show that a high-fat diet, as compared with a high-carb diet, is very effective at lowering levels of triglycerides, as long as the fats consumed are healthy.

Healthy fats actually purge the bad triglycerides and LDL from your bloodstream, thereby lowering the risk factors for heart disease. They clean up the blood

Increased energy

Insulin, which is secreted whenever carbs are consumed so that cells are able to absorb the energy, causes fatigue and drowsiness. This is why you often feel sleepy after eating a large meal. Additionally, glucose is not very efficient at creating energy and leaves a lot of waste products, thereby exacerbating fatigue. People on carb-rich diets tend to sleep much more than people on high-fat diets because they just don't have energy.

Once insulin levels are lowered and the body is adjusted to burning ketones instead of glucose, energy levels increase dramatically. Some people on the ketogenic diet report needing less sleep and are able to thrive on just six hours, whereas doctors recommend seven to eight. Interestingly, traditional cultures that consume high-fat diets also sleep closer to six hours, suggesting that there may be a link between eating a high-fat diet and needing less sleep.

Balanced hormones

At the heart of many diseases are imbalanced hormones. Insulin is one of the most proliferate hormones in the human body and problems with its levels immediately affect other hormones, including sex hormones, satiety hormones and hunger hormones. Stabilizing and permanently lowering insulin levels leads to balanced hormones all across the body. This is why people with metabolic syndrome, PCOS, acne and other hormonal problems benefit immensely from the ketogenic diet.

Decreased inflammation

Inflammation is the body's natural response to infection and foreign invaders. When you cut your finger, the skin around the cut quickly becomes red and inflamed, as your body is responding to the microbes that may be entering. While some inflammation is good as an acute response, many people live in a state of chronic inflammation caused by poor diet. Inflamed tissues can develop scar tissue and be unable to function properly. Inflamed joints become painful and inflamed blood vessels cause heart disease.

A ketogenic diet has been shown to substantially decrease inflammation over the long term. The body is still able to use inflammation as an acute response to foreign invaders, but it is no longer a chronic issue.

Chapter Four:
Basics of Planning Meals

To know what you have to eat on a ketogenic diet, you will have to understand caloric requirements and content and fats, protein and carbohydrates. You have to understand their different kinds and the different roles they perform for your body. Furthermore, you need to know what macronutrients are good and harmful for your health so that you can build a diet that is both ketogenic and healthy.

In addition, for the ketogenic diet to work, you need to remove all packaged and processed foods from your diet. It should consist of high-quality, healthy fats, fiber-rich carbohydrates with the least net carbohydrates (total carbohydrates minus fiber) as possible.

Important: Before you create a plan for your ketogenic diet, you need to consult first a nutritionist or a medical professional to determine the number of daily calories you require based on your age, height, weight, gender and age as well as body fat percentage. This would make sure that you are not merely guessing in setting the calories you need for your body.
Fats

In the 1980s, doctors, nutritionists and public health officials campaigned to the public that fats are not a part of a healthy diet. They said that fat is the cause of weight gain and heart disease. However, this is only true for the bad quality of fat in food. Fats play a critical role in providing a denser caloric content per gram compared to proteins and carbohydrates. Because of this, fat can provide adequate energy when food is scarce or when a person is unable to consume large amounts of food.

Fats

Fats in your diet contain mixtures of fatty acids. These nutrients contain a mixture of saturated and unsaturated fats. Saturated fats are most abundant in animal-derived fats while unsaturated fats are most abundant in plant-derived ones. Other than the dense caloric property fats, it provides fatty acids that regulate inflammation in the body. It carries fat-soluble vitamins. Lastly, it provides texture and flavor to your meal, making it more satisfying to your appetite.

Fats to avoid
Excess Saturated Fat

The key to having healthy fat consumption is to minimize the consumption of food rich in saturated fats. Although your body needs both kinds of fat, saturated fats from foods derived from plants are enough to provide you with your saturated fat needs. Having high levels of saturated fat in your body leads to heart and cardiovascular disease.

Moreover, it is not enough to replace saturated fat-rich foods with fat-free food products as these are high in carbohydrates and increase the risk of the same disease mentioned. Here's a list of foods rich in saturated fat that you should avoid:

- Fat from processed meats like sausages, ham and burgers

- Fatty meat
- Hard cheeses
- Butter
- Lard
- Ghee
- Palm Oil

Trans Fat

Trans fat, or trans-unsaturated fats, occur in nature albeit in small amounts, but they are also widely manufactured commercially from vegetable fats for use in various manufactured food products. This is created by adding hydrogen gas to vegetable oil, which causes the oil to become solid at room temperature.

The reason why food manufacturers create and use this is to make food have a longer shelf life or have a better flavor. These fats contribute to insulin resistance and unbalance your cholesterol levels by increasing the bad and decreasing the good.

Manufactured trans-fat can be found in food products like:

- Baked goods like cake, pie crusts and crackers and ready-made frosting
- Snacks like packaged microwave popcorn and potato, corn and tortilla chips.
- Fried food due to the oil used in the cooking process
- Refrigerator dough like canned biscuits, cinnamon rolls and frozen pizza crusts
- Non-dairy coffee creamer
- Margarine
- In food labels, trans fat can also be listed as shortening, hydrogenated oil, partially hydrogenated oil and hydrogenated vegetable oil.

Fats you can eat

The key to having a healthy ketogenic diet is choosing wisely the fats you include in your diet without exceeding your calorie requirement. The important part of this diet is to consume the correct ratio of macronutrients. You need between five and ten percent of your calories to be from net carbs, 15 and 30 percent from protein and 65 to 75 percent or more from fat to be able to benefit from the ketones that get produced by the liver.

Is there a right amount of fat intake with a ketogenic diet? This amount will vary for everybody. It depends on your goals. You don't need to count your calories or fat intake on a keto diet since eating foods that are naturally low in carbs keep your feeling full longer.

Studies have shown that fats and proteins are the most filling nutrients and carbs are the least. Fats contribute to a steady energy supply and don't cause insulin spikes. This is the reason you don't have cravings, mood swings or fluctuating energy. For some, counting calories and tracking macros can help break through a stubborn weight loss plateau.

The macronutrient ratio isn't all you need to consider. You need to understand what fats are good for you and what can be detrimental to your health. The different qualities and types of fat make a difference. When figuring out what fats and oil to use, here are some simple rules to follow:

When cooking, use saturated fats. These fats have gotten a bad rap as being bad for us. We have heard that cholesterol and saturated fats cause obesity and heart disease for the past 50 years. This lipid hypothesis was created by Ancel Keys' fraudulent and flawed research. Saturated fats can be found in palm oil, coconut oil, eggs, tallow, lard, ghee, butter, cream and red meat. These oils have a high smoke point, long shelf life and are the most stable. Use these for cooking. The majority of fats need to come from monounsaturated and saturated fats.

Try adding medium chain triglycerides to your diet. These are fats that can be easily digested. These triglycerides can be found in coconut oil. They act differently when ingested and are sent straight to the liver. They can be immediately used for energy. They are found in palm oil and butter in lesser quantities. Medium chain triglycerides are used by bodybuilders and athletes to improve their performance and help them lose fat. If your body is able to handle pure MCT oil without causing any stomach problems, you should be able to find it as a supplement.

Include monounsaturated fatty acids. Omega 9, oleic acid or monounsaturated fatty acids can be found in nuts, beef, olives and avocados. These help to prevent heart disease. Consuming

49

monounsaturated fatty acids can give better serum lipid profiles. Monounsaturated fatty acids like macadamia nut, avocado and extra virgin olive oil are the best for using cold like drizzling over a finished a meal.

You can use unsaturated fats. You do not heat them. Our body needs omega 6s, Omega 3s and polyunsaturated fatty acids. These are common in our everyday lives and we consume too many. These fatty acids are called poly because they have many double bonds. When these bonds are heated, they react with oxygen to form compounds that are harmful like free radicals. This process increases inflammation and makes free radicals that put us at risk for cancer and heart disease. Polyunsaturated fats are not stable and should not be used for high heat cooking. Avocado oil, flaxseed oil, sesame oil, nut oils and extra virgin olive oil are best to use cold. Flaxseed oil shouldn't be heated and needs to be refrigerated. Olive, Macadamia and avocado oil can be used for light cooking or for finishing the meal.

The Omega 6 fatty acids and omega 3 fatty acids need to be balanced. Both of these are polyunsaturated fatty acids and are essential. Studies have shown that most diets are deficient in omega 3s. The omega 6 and omega 3 ratio is unfavorable between 15 to 1 and 17 to 1. This ratio needs to be balanced at one to one. It will be better for your health if you can get this ratio as close to one to one as possible. Studies have shown that eating more omega 6 and lower omega 3s are known to cause inflammatory diseases, autoimmune disorders, stroke and cardiovascular disease. Reducing your intake of omega 6s might protect you against these diseases. You are probably getting enough omega 6s so try to focus on increasing the intake of omega 3s by eating macadamia nuts, walnuts, grass-fed meat, fermented cod liver oil and wild salmon.

Your Omega 3 intake should come from animals. Omega 3 is either long chain that is found in seafood and fish or short chain that is found in nuts and seeds. While Eicosapentaenoic acid or EPA and docosahexaenoic acid or DHA affect omega 6s to 3s ratios, the alpha-linoleic acid or ALA needs to be converted to DHA or EPA. Our bodies can't convert ALA to DHA or EPA. This is why you need to get the omega 3s from the meat of animals. When buying meat, find grass fed to get the most omega 3s. Meat from animals that have been grain fed had very low omega 3s but packed full of omega 6s.

Be aware of shelf life, oxidation rate and smoke point. A higher smoke point is better. Oils that have a high smoke point can be used to cook foods at high temperatures. If you heat the oil above its smoke point, this can damage the oil and release free radicals.

Having an oxidation rate that is slow is better. The oxidation rate increases when it gets heated to its smoking point. These can also oxidize on the shelf. Metals like copper and iron can also cause them to oxidize. Any oil is capable of going rancid while sitting on in the pantry. This will load them with free radicals. Higher saturated fat oils will last longer around 12 to 24 months. Oils that are high in monounsaturated fats will last about six to twelve months. Polyunsaturated fats have a shelf life of about two to six months.

Stay away from all unhealthy oils. Corn, grapeseed, soybean, canola, cottonseed, safflower, sunflower oils, trans fats, partially hydrogenated oils, hydrogenated oils, margarine and processed vegetable oils are all bad for your health. Processed oils and trans fatty acids:

- Are oxidized with high heat and created free radicals.
- These are created from genetically modified seeds.
- Are pro-inflammatory and bad for your gut.
- Eating trans fats raises the risk of developing coronary heart disease.

- Consuming trans fats will affect cholesterol levels negatively. They reduce the level of HDL or good cholesterol and increase the level of LDL or bad cholesterol.
- Can cause an increased risk of cancer.

All of these fats exist within nature and occur during the processing of polyunsaturated fatty acids in food production. These naturally occurring trans fats are beneficial when you compare them to artificial trans fats. These natural trans fats can be found in the meat of animals that have been grass fed and dairy products.

Metabolic poison refers to artificial trans fats. Get these out of your diet by staying away from any food that contains partially hydrogenated or hydrogenated oils. You can find these in French fries, crackers, cookies and margarine.

Proteins

Most foods contain some amount of protein including vegetables and grain. Foods that have substantial amounts of protein are meat from animals, dairy products, beans and nuts. It can provide energy for your body. However, it is not its primary purpose.

When broken down into amino acids, the body would use this to create its own proteins intended for various purposes. With the 20 amino acids that your body would need, it can create an infinite number of proteins like enzymes for chemical reactions, hormones for triggering organs, collagen for bone structure and antibodies for the immune system. Your body's proteins are constantly broken down and re-synthesized to build more proteins. Most of the amino acids from broken down protein are reused, but some are lost and must be replaced through your diet.

Proteins to avoid

What you have to watch out for in proteins in your diet is eating too much of it. The excess protein that you got from your food would be converted to sugar and then fat which would be stored for later use. It could also increase the stimulation of your mTOR, which increases your chances of developing cancer. Additionally, the excess protein requires your body to remove more nitrogen, a by-product of protein digestion, which stresses out your kidneys.

Proteins to eat

Moderate consumption of high-quality protein is the key. Protein for a ketogenic diet should come from a variety of plant and animal sources. Meat products should be lean to avoid adding fats that are mostly saturated. The suggested protein for a ketogenic diet varies from person to person. Generally, the recommended daily protein of 0.8g per pound of lean body mass for a sedentary lifestyle, 0.8 to 1g per pound of body mass for a lightly active lifestyle and 1.0 – 1.2g for a highly active lifestyle.

Carbohydrates

Carbohydrates are the starches, sugars and fibers found in the food that we eat. The sugars and starches we eat are broken down into its simplest chemical forms while, as it is indigestible, fibers just pass through the digestive system.

Sugars, also known as simple carbohydrates, are found in fruit and vegetables that can be broken down to sucrose and/ or fructose. Starches, also known as complex carbohydrates, are found in grains that can be broken down into glucose (also known as blood sugar).

Of all these carbohydrates, glucose is the most preferred as it can be readily circulated from the digestive process into various parts of the body. Meanwhile, fructose can only be used for energy by the liver and sucrose is further broken down into glucose and fructose.

The role of fiber: The most common question with low carb dieters is: Do I need to include fiber when counting my carbs?

Let's see: Some soluble gets absorbed, but humans, in general, don't possess all the needed enzymes to digest fibers and then be able to get calories out of it. Because of this, fiber doesn't affect blood sugar or ketosis. You can try to get between 20 and 25 grams of net carbs or less than 50 grams of total carbs.

If the fiber isn't counted, the carbs are referred to as net carbs. Calculating net carbs can reduce how high fiber foods are impacted and allow you to eat them. This is a common argument for those who criticize the low carb diet because it lacks fiber. An important note is that fiber does not negate carbs. They are just not counted. You can't just mix some flax meal into pasta.

In Canada and the United States, food labels include fiber with the carbohydrate values in a term known as total carbs. This calculates carbs by using an indirect method. Carbs get calculated after the ash, water, fat and protein has been measured out. To figure net carbs, you subtract the amount of fiber from the total carbs. This type of food label isn't used all over the world. In Oceania, Australia and Europe, their food labels don't include fiber. They calculate carbs using a direct method. The carbs listed on their food labels will just be net carbs. Don't worry about where you buy the food but think about the country it came from.

Is there a way to be certain about the amounts of net carbs? You can follow these rules:

- Total carbs will never be less than the amount of fiber.
- The total carbs minus the fiber is never going to be less than the sugar. For example, lactose + other sugar + sugars = net carbs.
- Calories that come from carbs (without fiber) + calories that come from protein + calories that come from fat

= total kcal

Although fiber cannot be digested, it plays a key role in the digestion of carbohydrates in the body. It slows down the rate of digestion and absorption of carbohydrates, thereby preventing the blood sugar from rapidly shooting up. Aside from that, fibers provide food for your beneficial gut bacteria, improving digestion and bowel movement.

Fibers also contain phytochemicals like lycopene, lutein and indole-3-carbinol. These stimulate the immune system, fight free radicals and protect and repair the DNA.

Carbs to avoid

Refined Carbohydrates

Refined carbohydrates are whole plants or plant-derived products that have been processed to remove everything except the highly digestible carbohydrate in it. To refine carbohydrates, the whole sugar, plant, or grain is stripped of its fibers, vitamins and minerals. This is done usually as other parts of the plant cannot be digested by the body or to make the plant easier to manipulate into mixtures and food products.

Refining removes everything including valuable natural vitamins and minerals and, to circumvent the lack of micronutrients, manufacturers add synthetic vitamins and minerals back into the carbohydrates.

Refined carbohydrates in an average person's diet usually come from:

- White flour from white bread, pasta and other food products containing it.
- White rice that is usually "enriched" with the synthetic vitamins and minerals.
- Sugar from bread, pastries, sweets and breakfast cereals.
- Sugar and High Fructose Corn Syrup from sodas and other sweetened beverages.
- Sugar from any other food product that has been added before consumption like ketchup and mustard.

With the fibers removed from these carbohydrates, your body digests it quickly. This results in a rapid absorption of broken down carbohydrates into your body. Particularly, in the case of glucose, your blood sugar rises so fast that your body would have to release insulin to signal your body to start storing it. This causes a volatile and erratic volume of blood sugar in your system. This usually manifests to sluggishness and/ or hunger even though you just had a heavy carbohydrate meal. If your body experiences this often, it will pave the way for insulin resistance and, eventually, Type 2 Diabetes.

On the other hand, fructose from refined carbohydrates that are used as sweeteners and other forms of added sugars have compound said harmful effects. Excess consumption of foods containing added fructose could lead to:

- Visceral fat gain
- Increased uric acid levels leading to gout and high blood pressure,
- Insulin resistance
- Leptin resistance that disturbs body fat regulation and contributing to obesity.

High Fructose Corn Syrup

High Fructose Corn Syrup (HFCS) is a refined carbohydrate that comes from corn. It is a sugar substitute that is a hundred times sweeter than sucrose, the common sugar. Since it costs substantially less and is not affected by fluctuating import prices, it is a very good alternative for sugar. It started gaining popularity during the 1970s when it began being used by food manufacturers. Its use in different food products steadily rose since then.

The incidences of obesity are higher in countries where its use is prevalent. Add to that the fact, that in the 1980s up to the present date, obesity rates in the United States steadily rose, matching the trend of rising availability of HFCS in food products.

Moreover, studies have shown that, even in moderate consumption, HFCS is a major cause of various diseases like heart disease, obesity, cancer, dementia and liver failure. Even though HFCS is used as a substitute for sucrose, the body does not respond to it in the same way.

Carbs to Eat

In a ketogenic diet, you must stick to protein, vegetables, fats and oils, full-fat dairy and nuts and seeds of your diet. From these items, you will already be able to get the fiber that you need for your diet. Adding any kind of grain or sugar in your diet would only prevent you from reaching your goals in the diet. However, if you want to have your fix of carbohydrates, you can use flour substitutes like coconut flour and flaxseed meal.

For carbohydrates in a Standard Ketogenic Diet, the maximum daily intake is 5% of total daily calorie intake. Refer to the net carbs of the food items given in preparing the carbohydrates for your meals.

Beverages

The ketogenic diet is very particular in controlling what goes into your body. Drinking alcohol, sweetened beverages and fruit juices would mess up your sugar levels and could push you further from reaching ketosis. Therefore, you must only drink water and coffee and tea with no sweeteners, creamer and dairy. Anything else other than these three should not be drunk.

The ketogenic diet causes a natural diuretic effect. Dehydration is common for many people who are just starting on this diet. If you get bladder pain or urinary tract infections, you need to be prepared. The normal eight glasses that are recommended for you to drink - you need to drink those and then more. Our body consists of two-thirds water. Drink at least a gallon of water everyday, as hydration is extremely important.

Many choose keto friendly coffee or tea of the mornings to give their energy a boost with added fats. It is good; just remember to avoid flavored beverages as much as possible. This becomes amplified with caffeine as too much may hamper your weight loss. Try to only have about two caffeinated beverages each day.

Some examples of beverages you can have with your keto diet are:

- Water: This is your go-to for hydration. You may have sparkling or plain water.
- Broth: This is loaded with nutrients and vitamins. Most important, it gives your energy a boost by replenishing your electrolytes.
- Coffee: This will improve your mental focus and has weight loss benefits.
- Tea: This has the same effects as coffee. Some people don't like tea. Try either green or black tea.
- Almond or coconut milk: Use the unsweetened versions in a carton from your grocery store to replace your favorite dairy drink.
- Diet soda: You need to reduce or completely stop drinking these. These can cause sugar cravings and insulin spikes.
- Flavoring: These little packets are flavored with stevia or sucralose and are fine. You can also add orange, lime and lemon to your water.
- Alcohol: If you need your alcohol, choose hard liquor. Wine and beer will be too high in carbs to drink. Frequent consumption of alcohol will slow down your weight loss.

Most people like to keep themselves accountable for the actions by creating a challenge for themselves. Try using a 32-ounce water bottle and place four hair-ties around it. Every time you finish a bottle, take away one hair tie. Keep on drinking until there aren't any left.

Recommended Foods

Below is a comprehensive list of the common food items that are recommended for your ketogenic diet. Each item has information of its nutritional value arranged as such: "amount of item/ calories/fat / net carbohydrates/protein."

Protein

The best proteins for a ketogenic diet are those that are pasture-raised and grass-fed. This will minimize your exposure from bacteria and growth hormones. Choose darker poultry meat and fatty fish that are rich in omega 3. Balance out your protein portions in your meals with fats and oil to aid in its digestion.

- Ground beef (4oz, 80/ 20 / 280 / 23g / 0g / 20g)
- Ribeye steak (4oz / 330 / 25g / 0g / 27g)
- Bacon (4oz / 519 / 51g / 0g / 13g)
- Pork chop (4oz / 286 / 18g / 0g / 30g)
- Chicken thigh (4oz / 250 / 20g / 0g / 17g)
- Chicken breast (4oz / 125 / 1g / 0 / 26g)
- Salmon (4oz / 236 / 15g / 0g / 23g)
- Ground lamb (4oz / 319 / 27g / 0g / 19g)
- Liver (4oz / 135 / 5g / 0g / 19g)
- Egg (1 large / 70 / 5g / 0.5g / 6g)
- Almond butter (2tbsp / 180 / 16g / 4g/ 6)

Vegetables and Fruit

Cruciferous vegetables that are grown above ground, leafy and green are the best for a ketogenic diet. On the other hand, vegetables that grow below ground should be eaten in moderation as these have higher carbohydrate amounts.

- Cabbage (6 oz. / 43g / 0g / 6g / 2g)
- Cauliflower (6 oz. / 40 / 0g / 6g / 5g)
- Broccoli (6 oz. / 58 / 1g / 7g / 5g)
- Spinach (6 oz. / 24 / 0g / 1g / 3g)
- Romaine Lettuce (6 oz. / 29 / 1g / 2g / 2g)
- Green Bell Pepper (6 oz. / 33 / 0g / 5g / 1g)
- Baby Bella Mushrooms (6 oz. / 40 / 0g / 4g / 6g)
- Green Beans (6 oz. / 26 / 0g / 4g / 2g)
- Yellow Onion (6 oz. / 68 / 0g / 12g/ 2g)
- Blackberries (6 oz. / 73 / 1g / 8g / 2g)
- Raspberries (6 oz. / 88 / 1g / 8g / 2g)

Dairy Products

If available, give preference to raw and organic dairy products. Avoid highly processed dairy as these have a higher amount of carbohydrates than raw/ organic ones. Also avoid products with higher carbohydrate levels.

- Heavy cream (1 oz. / 100g / 12g / 0g / 0g)
- Greek yogurt (1 oz. / 28g / 1g / 1g / 3g)
- Mayonnaise (1 oz. / 180g / 20g / 0g / 0g)
- Half n' half (1 oz. / 40 / 4g / 1g / 1g)
- Cottage cheese (1 oz. / 25g / 1g / 1g / 4g)
- Cream Cheese (1 oz. / 94 / 9g / 1g / 2g)
- Mascarpone (1 oz. / 120g / 13g / 0g / 2g)
- Mozzarella (1 oz. / 70 / 5g / 1g / 5g)
- Brie (1 oz. / 95 / 8g / 0g / 6g)
- Aged Cheddar (1 oz. / 110 / 9g / 0g / 7g)

- Parmesan (1 oz. / 110 / 7g / 1g / 10g)

Nuts and Seeds

These are best when roasted to remove any anti-nutrients present. These can be added to add flavor or texture to your meals.

- Macadamia Nuts (2 oz. / 407 / 43g / 3g / 4g)
- Brazil Nuts (2 oz. / 373 / 37g / 3g / 8g)
- Pecans (2 oz. / 392 / 41g / 3g / 5g)
- Almonds (2 oz. / 328 / 28g / 5g / 12g)
- Hazelnuts (2 oz. / 356 / 36g / 3g / 9g)

Nut and Seed Flours

These can be used as a substitute for regular flour in making baked and dessert recipes.

- Almond Flour (2 oz. / 324 / 28g / 6g / 12g)
- Coconut Flour (2 oz. / 120 / 4g / 6g / 4g)
- Chia Seed Meal (2 oz. / 265 / 17g / 3g / 8g)
- Flaxseed Meal (2 oz. / 224 / 18g / 1g / 8g)
- Unsweetened Coconut (2 oz. / 445 / 40g / 8g / 4g)

Getting Started

Before you even get started on this diet, you must first decide on your goal and why you're doing this. Are you looking to lose unhealthy body fat? Are you looking to therapeutically heal a degenerative disease? Are you aiming to change your lifestyle? Whatever the case may be, you must first decide why you're going to do this diet. Without clarity on your goal, you can't choose an approach for your diet and can't properly plan for how to do it.

Get Yourself Tested

You must first determine that your body can undergo the diet and the massive adjustments it would make. You also have to determine your body fat percentage, weight and other relevant data to create your personal macronutrient mix via keto calculators available online.

Get Support

You have to talk to your family, especially if they live in the same house as you. If you're the only one who's doing this diet, your family might misunderstand when you can't eat like them, or you have a different food from theirs. Moreover, on the first few weeks, you might miss out on the next birthday party or family gathering just to distance yourself from tempting carbohydrates.

Other than that, your family can also help you in keeping you in line with the diet. They can call you out whenever you're about to slip from it. Also, if you have children, you can make it fun for them by making them your carbohydrate police at home. If you live alone, you can get support by joining community forums online.

Plan the meals that you will have

Even before you shop for your ketogenic groceries, you must first know the meals you will be eating beforehand. This would save you time and would make sure that you have the right ingredients ready for making ketogenic meals. This would reduce the excuses you can think of to just nibble on carbohydrates or say, "it would just be one meal."

Also, this gives you the opportunity to research for recipes that you might like. Other than that, after you find recipes that you like, you can plan out your meals for your next run to the grocery. Clean out the Carbohydrates out of Your House

This is the best way of preventing yourself from slipping up and "accidentally" eating that cookie. If there are no food items in your house to tempt you, you cannot be tempted to eat what you shouldn't. This would surely help you, as the first few months are the hardest due to your body still adapting to ketosis.

Undergo an Adaptation Period

To make the ketogenic diet easier for you, you could slowly ease into it by either fasting intermittently to or cut your carbohydrates. By fasting intermittently, you have 16 hours wherein you don't eat anything and only 8 hours wherein you can. This forces your body to enter a state of fasting and you get used to having your blood sugar into a fasted state.

On the other hand, by cutting your calories, your body is being trained to get used to having smaller portions of carbohydrates that it used to. Like in intermittent fasting, it decreases the shock of having very little carbohydrates in your diet. One practice is by limiting daily net carbohydrates to only 30 grams for 6 days in a week and having a high carbohydrate meal for dinner of the 7th day. This is repeated for every 7 days for at least 4 weeks.

Chapter Five:
Setting up a Plan

I n this section, I will familiarize you with some practical aspects that you might need to know about to set up a plan.

Keto Shopping List

There are plenty of keto foods out there. Here is a list to help you get started with your first shopping trip:

Vegetables:

- Asparagus
- Broccoli
- Cabbage
- Pickles
- Black Olives
- Green Olives
- Sauerkraut
- Cauliflower
- Spinach, fresh and canned
- Green onions
- Iceberg Lettuce
- Mushrooms
- Okra
- Spaghetti Squash
- Yellow Onions

- Zucchini
- Yellow Squash
- Leeks
- Canned Green Beans

Fruit:

- Any berry
- Rhubarb
- Tomatoes in moderation
- Lemons
- Limes
- Avocado
- Coconut
- Figs
- Watermelon
- Cherries
- Pomegranate
- Papaya
- Raisins
- Plums
- Clementine
- Apple
- Guava

Dairy:

- Full Fat Milk
- Full Fat Greek Yogurt
- Mayonnaise
- Heavy Whipping Cream
- Sour Cream

Cheeses:

- Swiss
- String Cheese
- Parmesan
- Mozzarella
- Monterey Jack
- Goat Cheese
- Feta
- Cream Cheese
- Cottage Cheese
- Colby
- Cheddar
- Brie
- Blue

Meats:

- Beef
- Chicken
- Pork
- Turkey
- Tuna
- Salmon
- Cod
- Flounder
- Tilapia
- Shrimp
- Scallops
- Lobster

Spices:

- All herbs and spices

Dressings and Sauces:

- Lime Juice
- Lemon Juice
- Italian
- Ranch
- Blue Cheese
- Brown and Yellow Mustard
- Worcestershire Sauce
- Vinegar
- Soy Sauce
- Sugar-Free Syrup
- Sugar-Free Ketchup
- Low-Carb Salsa

Liquids:

- Protein Shakes
- Unsweetened Tea
- Coffee (can add heavy cream)
- Almond Milk
- Cashew Milk
- Coconut Milk

Oils and Fats:

- Sunflower Oil
- Sesame Oil
- Peanut Oil

- Olive Oil
- Mayonnaise
- Coconut Oil
- Bacon Fat
- Butter

Baking and Cooking:

- Cocoa Power
- Chia Seeds
- Flax Seeds
- Flax Meal
- Almond Meal/Flour
- Coconut Flakes
- Coconut Flour

Sweeteners:

- Xylitol
- Stevia Drops
- Erythritol

Evaluate Your Keto Diet Experience

With your meal plan and recipes ready to go and your mind ready for the diet, you begin. In the first week, things immediately start to get uncomfortable and your energy seems to have dropped to almost nonexistent levels. This shouldn't come as a surprise since this is normal for anyone and it is simply signs of your body being in a transition.

Common Side Effects

With any change to your diet, it is normal to have some side effects as your body begins to adapt to the new way you are eating. When doing a ketogenic diet, the body must switch the fuel source from glucose to fat stores. This can cause some of the following side effects:

Keto Flu

With your body used to only breaking down carbohydrates and using it for energy, it had built up numerous enzymes dedicated to this process. Because of the body's dependence on carbohydrates, it neglected the production of enzymes for dealing with fats. Then, your body is suddenly dealing with a lack of glucose and constant supply of fats, which triggers the body to start producing enzymes for using fat as fuel.

However, this would take time and not only one or two days. The first few weeks on a keto diet is challenging for some and easy for others. Your body is used to relying on glucose for energy, so it needs to switch to using ketones for fuel. This can result in brain fog but disappears when the body gets adapted. This adaptation takes about four weeks, but the side effects disappear sooner. Around the end of the first week, it is normal to feel some flu-like symptoms like cravings, insomnia, racing heart when lying down, fatigue, dizziness and brain fog. You can lessen these effects by gradually lowering your carb intake over a few weeks. If you decide to just right into a keto diet, just remember to get plenty of fluids and salts. This will keep you from feeling lousy.

This is called Keto Flu and is a natural transitional response of your body. This usually happens during the first week of your ketogenic diet. In this state, you will experience headaches, mental fogginess, dizziness and aggravation. These ailments are due to your electrolytes being eliminated in your body because ketones have a diuretic effect. To counteract this, you should drink plenty of water and increase the sodium in your body.

<u>Curing the Keto Flu</u>

The keto flu will vary with each person. Many find the symptoms are worst in the first week. Some find they linger for weeks on end. There are some tricks you can do to shorten your flu time:

- Eat more fats: This is a common method used to combat the keto flu. Your body needs energy. It isn't getting it from sugar and carbs, so it needs to get it from what you are eating. Eat lots of healthy fats like lard, tallow, ghee, olive oil and coconut oil. To stay in ketosis, you need to consume plenty of fats. Adding MCT oil can boost your ketone level. This will help your brain feel better.
- Eat more calories: It is easy to not eat enough when you begin a low carb diet. Many just cut out the carbs without increasing other food intakes. They get confused about what they can eat since they are used to eating bread, rice and pasta.
- Exercise: This might be the last thing you are thinking about right now. Studies show that exercise helps you to become more metabolically flexible. This means that your body can switch between carbs and ketones for energy easily. People that don't experience the keto flu for long are more metabolically flexible because they can switch between ketones and carbs.

Bad Breath

This is sometimes called keto breath. It can happen as you go into ketosis. Ketones get released into the breath, sweat and urine. Acetone is one form of a ketone that is released in the breath and can cause a metallic taste in the mouth. This is temporary and will disappear after a couple of weeks. If this becomes a problem, sugar-free breath fresheners or gum can help. You can increase your oral hygiene by using mouthwash and brushing your teeth more often.

Leg Cramps

Developing muscle cramps might be possible with the keto diet. These can sometimes be rather bothersome. The cause of cramps is a condition called hyponatremia. This happens when salt levels are too low. Stay hydrated and add salt to the diet.

Loss of Salts

There will be changes in your fluid balance in the first few weeks on the keto diet. This happens as the body uses up the stored sugars that in turn release water into the blood that gets flushed out through the urine. When fluids get passed out, salts in the body will become depleted. Keep yourself hydrated. Water is best, but coffee and tea are fine as long as they aren't extremely milky. Make sure you have plenty of salt, so you won't experience side effects like wooziness and headaches. You can add sea salt to your food and drink bone or vegetable bouillons and broths. Magnesium and potassium are important salts, too.

If you are eating natural, healthy foods like vegetables, dairy, fish, meat and nuts, you shouldn't have any problems getting the potassium and magnesium you need.

Bowel Habit Change

A keto diet can cause constipation. The body's gut bacteria need to adapt to be able to handle the different foods and the different amounts of food. Bowel habits usually improve in a couple of weeks. If they don't, make sure you are getting enough fiber. Drink lots of water and increase the amounts of seeds, nuts, legumes and fibrous vegetables.

Loss of Energy

The biggest misconception of the keto diet is the lack of glucose will deplete the body of its energy. Keeping steady energy is more challenging with a standard diet because it fluctuates with blood sugar.

Eating lower carbs doesn't prevent the sugar level rollercoaster. Once the body gets into ketosis, the body begins to draw energy from its fat stores. The liver begins to create the amount of glucose the body needs.

By cutting down on carbs, the body will find it easier to regulate energy and sugar level. You might notice a dip in energy while adapting to the diet; this should pass in a few weeks.

Poor Physical Performance

Due to low levels of blood sugar, your physical performance will drop. This is only for the short term and your body will eventually adapt to it. However, if you have to always be on top of your performance, it will be beneficial for you if you adopt either the Cyclic or Targeted Ketogenic Diet. These two approaches will provide you the energy for your physical activities and, at the same time, enable you to have a ketogenic diet.

Other than that, you may also experience cramps, constipation and heart palpitations. These are easily remedied by your proper hydration and by eating foods with good sources of micronutrients. There is nothing to be alarmed when you experience these effects. In fact, they tell you that your body is adjusting to a state of ketosis.

These side effects are normally temporary and can be remedied.

Signs that you've reached Ketosis
- Bad breath due to acetone, a ketone being expelled through your mouth or urine.
- Dry mouth and increased thirst due to ketones being diuretics.
- Increased urination

What to watch out for

It is important to keep track of your ketones to make sure that your body is responding to the diet and to prevent ketoacidosis. It is when the ketones in your body approach dangerous levels. Although it is easy to assume that ketones can reach high levels, this is simply not true and is, in fact, a rare occurrence.

It is still important to regularly keep track of your ketones. This can easily be done and no need for laboratory tests to be done. Ketone testing can easily be done through urine strips, breath ketone analyzers and blood ketone meter.

Keeping up Motivation

Beginning a new diet is exciting. You see all the transformation pictures online and you start to see how your body will change, also. Sticking to a keto diet until it becomes your lifestyle gets challenging. If you can stick to the keto diet for a few months, you will get the results of more energy, mental clarity and loss of body fat. Here are some techniques to help you:

1. Start small. It is tempting to go all in in the beginning. Your motivation will be high and we have a tendency to push ourselves to the limit. We think we have to cook all our meals at home instead of going out to eat. We

have to join a gym and work out for hours five days a week. This will cause the body to crash and burn and the result is stopping the diet completely. The answer to this is the pick a small change that is easy to commit to. If you want to change your whole diet, start by changing your breakfast. Don't go to the gym for hours every day just do 15 minutes two times a week. By starting small, it will be impossible not to do it. Create the habit first and then increase it once you have gained traction.

2. Eat the same things. The reason many people don't stick to a diet is that they are looking for a variety each day. If they get stressed out or their willpower is tested, they just go to a fast food restaurant. If they can learn to eat the same meals each day, it will reduce the likelihood of cheating since you already know what you are going to eat. Repeat the same three or four meal over and over. Try variety on the weekends.

3. Take some food with you. We might not always be around keto friendly food. It might be a family gathering or a party at work. The temptation is everywhere. The key here is controlling your environment. Pack a lunchbox or backpack full of keto-friendly snacks to take with you wherever you go. If you begin to feel tempted grab a handful and eat away. This might save you from cheating on your diet.

4. Make success rewarding. Most people know how to lose weight. Having a true reason to change is the answer, not more information. Use positive reinforcements to help. Set realistic weight loss goals for yourself like losing ten pounds in 30 days. Think of something that you have wanted to do for a long time like taking a trip someplace you've never been or spending the day at a spa. You can only do this if you reach your weight loss goal.

5. Never try to be perfect. Stay focused on the progress, not perfection. Be okay with grabbing a non-keto snack every now and then. Too many have

quit reaching for their goal because they think they have failed. We are all human. To err is human. The real failure here is just giving up.

Long-Term Tips

No matter how much you love the ketogenic diet, there are family reunions, parties and other events that can easily derail your best-laid plans. Holidays and birthdays can be particularly difficult, as you are surrounded by sweet and savory dishes that bring back fond memories. Being surrounded by relatives and friends who lovingly prepared all of the food can make resisting even more difficult. Having to prepare food separately from what you feed your family can be difficult. Additionally, you are probably finding that the ketogenic diet takes a lot of commitment. Food preparation, storage and grocery shopping can take vastly larger amounts of time than before. Plus, it costs more than eating a high-carb diet. Here are some tips to help you stay on the ketogenic diet long-term.

Plan ahead

Planning your meals in advance is a strategic way to manage a busy schedule while sticking to a healthy eating plan. Prepare your grocery list before you go to the store so that you don't forget anything that you need. Having to make an extra grocery trip during the week can easily cost you an hour or two.

Make sure that you always have keto-friendly foods on you. Invest in some food containers that you can easily put in your bag and take with you places. Keep them filled with things like nuts, vegetable sticks, yogurt dip and sliced avocados. At a sports game, in a meeting, out on a long shopping excursion, or anytime that you have to be away from home for more than a few hours, you can pop the containers out and recharge on ketogenic foods.

One challenge of the ketogenic diet is that many foods have to be eaten immediately after being prepared. The thought of eating scrambled eggs that have been in the refrigerator for a couple of days is less than appetizing. Look for recipes that can be prepared in advance and eaten throughout the week. Examples include curries, soups and casseroles. Take one day each week to prepare some dishes that can be refrigerated and eaten throughout the week. This will save you a lot of time and enable you to stay on track, even on your busiest days.

Know what local restaurants have keto-friendly options on their menus so that when you do go out to eat, you already know what you can order without derailing your diet. Just because something isn't labeled keto-friendly doesn't mean that it isn't. An omelet with cheese is probably fine, as long as you don't add hash browns or anything else on the side. If you are at a restaurant that doesn't have anything that appears to be keto-friendly, ask for something to be specially prepared, based on the ingredients that appear in the other foods on the menu. For example, if there are choices that contain avocados, cucumbers and oil and vinegar dressing, you can request that those ingredients be made into a salad.\

Take advantage of grocery delivery

Grocery shopping can be a time-consuming hassle, but nowadays, many stores offer grocery delivery. You select online what you want and when you want it to be delivered, then pay online via credit or debit card. This can shave hours every week off of the time you spend on maintaining your keto diet.

Keep in mind that grocery delivery usually carries a fee and may be more expensive than going to the store, so make sure that you are aware of the cost. If you live in a large city, there may be several different stores that offer grocery delivery that you can check out.

Let others know of your diet

Before going out with friends or going to visit relatives, let them know that you are on the ketogenic diet. Inform them that you don't expect them to prepare any special food for you but that there are many foods that you will not be able to eat. Try to select restaurants that you know have keto-friendly options so that you and your friends can enjoy eating whatever you prefer. And who knows? You may find that others want to join you on the ketogenic diet!

Make friends with others who are on the ketogenic diet

Joining a group of people who are already on the ketogenic diet can be a great way to achieve accountability with people who are working towards the same goals. People who have already been where you are can give you practical advice about how they dealt with the side effects of adjusting to the diet and a state of ketosis, as well as how to handle things like the holidays and those worried emails from your parents about the supposed dangers of going keto. They can also give you pointers about things like saving money on groceries and cooking keto meals separately from what your family normally eats.

While you should avoid preaching to your friends about going keto, some may see how much the diet has benefited you and want to join in. You can hook them up with your buddies who are already on the ketogenic diet and work together as accountability partners.

Exercise regularly

The benefits of exercise are so immense that it is a wonder that doctors don't prescribe it instead of medication. It boosts immunity, improves blood flow and circulation, elevates mood, increases metabolism, burns off the stress hormones that can accumulate after traumatic events or as part of a hectic daily life, burns calories, purges blood sugar, relieves constipation, reduces insulin, the list goes on and on. One reason nutritionists may be against the ketogenic diet is that it doesn't necessarily incorporate exercise.

Commonly, people get onto the ketogenic diet as a shortcut to losing weight instead of as part of a healthy lifestyle, which has to include exercise. If you go onto the ketogenic diet, it needs to be because you want to improve your health, not just because you want to lose weight. Losing weight is a side effect of increased health and wellness. You need to exercise for at least thirty minutes four times a week.

Going for a brisk walk in the evening or for a morning jog is a great way to get started with exercise. Taking the stairs instead of the elevator and parking further away from the store instead of fighting for a front-row parking spot are easy ways to incorporate exercise into your daily life. You may want to join a gym or buy in-home exercise equipment, but you don't have to. Most people who buy gym membership or exercise equipment never use it unless they were already exercising regularly beforehand.

The best way to make exercise a meaningful and regular part of your life is to make it enjoyable. Put on some music and listen to your favorite songs while you are running on the treadmill. Go for a walk with your family or a friend. You will soon find that you feel so much better, both physically and emotionally, that you will want to continue exercising as much as possible.

Plan keto nights with friends

Your friends and/or family don't understand the ketogenic diet and they frequently discourage you from following it. Your mom repeatedly sends you emails with articles about how dangerous the ketogenic diet is and your best friend keeps tempting you with your favorite carb-rich foods to try to get you to start eating "normally" again. They have no idea why you would spend so much time preparing high-fat meals at home. So show them!

Plan keto nights in which you prepare keto-friendly foods for your friends and family to try. Have all of the ingredients out and enlist their help to prepare the meal. They might find themselves pleasantly surprised at how appetizing the ketogenic diet really is and some might even decide to join you!

Drink lots of water

Because the water-rich foods that you probably once enjoyed, like mangoes and apples, are no longer staples in your diet, you are consuming significantly less water than before. Additionally, when you are first starting out on the ketogenic diet, your kidneys will have to work harder to process all of the fat you are consuming along with the glucose and glycogen stores that your body is burning through. You will have to be intentional about drinking a lot of water. You will probably need to drink one ounce for every pound of body weight. If you are 160 pounds, you will probably need 160 ounces of water per day.

Practice intermittent fasting

Intermittent fasting is the practice of fasting for between 16 and 48 hours at a time for the purpose of gaining health benefits. Intermittent fasting has numerous health benefits. It turns on your body's fat burning processes, improves mental clarity and gets you into a state of ketosis.

You naturally are going into a fasting state at night when you sleep, because you aren't eating. Intermittent fasting extends this state throughout the day. Some experts prescribe fasts as a prelude to beginning the ketogenic diet and others advise fasts as a way to get the most benefits out of it. This is actually much easier than you may think because the ketogenic diet leads to significantly less hunger. When fasting, make sure that you consume plenty of fluids. You may want to supplement with things like coconut oil and butter to help induce ketosis.

Decrease your stress levels

Many of us live hectic, stressful lives. We are busy from the time we wake up until we go to sleep and increasing demands are constantly placed on us. You may find that you are constantly stressed to please your boss at work, care for your children and/or aging parents, maintain your home, keep up with finances, the list goes on and on. Our use of smartphones keeps us constantly connected, which can easily mean that the boss expects us to be readily available to answer emails and phone calls after hours. With today's tough economy, you may find that you are working a lot of extra hours or even two jobs (or more!) to try to stay afloat financially. Just let it be said that stress is an epidemic and you are probably not immune to it.

The effects of stress can be disastrous for anyone's health. In response to stress, the body releases cortisol and adrenaline and induces a "fight or flight" response. Many people actually live in a perpetual fight-or-flight state and are unable to shut their minds down, even to be able to sleep at night. The cortisol causes fat to build up in the abdominal area, which is the most harmful place for fat to accumulate. Stress also causes blood pressure to rise and increases the risk of other heart diseases. It easily makes people irritable, causing harmful effects on their relationships. Mood disorders, like depression and anxiety, can develop. Chronic stress can also lead to autoimmune problems, digestive issues, insomnia, skin problems like eczema and acne, infertility and cognitive issues. It can also inhibit a state of ketosis because stress hormones actually raise blood sugar and insulin and drive down ketone production. Needless to say, reducing stress is an important step in maintaining a healthy lifestyle.

Think about what you can reasonably do to decrease the stress in your life. You may need to take major steps, like considering a job change or lowering your hours at work. You may need to make other small changes, like reducing your financial obligations or turning off your smartphone at certain hours. Many people find that working with a counselor to help them deal with the toxic effects of stress and identify its causes is very beneficial in improving their quality of life.

You may be going through a particularly stressful or even traumatic period in your life. If that is the case, maintaining a state of ketosis may not be a reasonable goal. Instead, aim to eat a low-carb, high-fat diet, exercise regularly and seek out support from family, friends and possibly a professional.

Monitor your health

Because the ketogenic diet induces so many chemical changes in your body's metabolism, you need to keep tabs on different markers of health. You can easily buy ketone-testing strips that measure your ketone production through breath, blood, or urine. The ketogenic diet tends to reduce the electrolytes in your body, so you may want to get a tool that measures electrolytes in order to ensure you have an adequate amount. Because the goal of the ketogenic diet is ultimately to suppress the use of glucose for energy by inducing ketosis, you may want to get some tools for testing your blood sugar and insulin levels. These tools are easily available, as they are frequently used by diabetics as part of their daily regimens.

There are easy ways to monitor whether or not you are dehydrated. If your urine is yellow, cloudy and/or has a strong odor, you are probably dehydrated and need to drink a lot of water. This can also mean that you are drinking enough fluids but not enough water, so cut back on things like milk, coffee and tea and replace them with water. Another dehydration test is to pinch your arm. If the skin immediately snaps back into place, you are fine. If it sags or takes a moment to return to its original position, then you are dehydrated.

If implemented correctly, the ketogenic diet can become a lifelong lifestyle of health and wellness that will improve your wellbeing for years to come.

Mistakes to Avoid

Now let's look at the top mistakes Keto Dieters make and strategies to overcome them. It is helpful to keep them in mind even after you are successfully leading a Keto Lifestyle.

Mistake 1: Not Knowing your Macro Proportions

Ketosis is a reversible phenomenon. So long as you are using fat as your primary food and burning ketones for energy you will be able to control your weight and blood sugar levels. As soon you switch back to carbs, eat too much of proteins or reduce the proportion of fat in your diet, the body goes back to burning sugar for energy.

That's why maintaining an optimum proportion of Fats, Proteins and Carbs in your diet is so important for a Ketogenic Diet. Majority of the people falter in keeping this balance of proportion in a sustainable way over a long period of time.

<u>So what is the Optimum Proportion?</u>

Again, the answer to this question is more nuanced than you would like to hear. In short, the answer is, Know Your Own Body. Please find the recommended ranges below, but you will have to work with your body to determine the optimum amounts suitable to keep you in Ketosis.

In terms of percentage ratio the following proportions are recommended:

- Fat 60-75%
- Protein 15-30%
- Carbs 5-10%

Broadly the proportion depends on the following factors:

- Your Body Mass Index
- Your Age
- Your Percentage Body Fat
- Your Activity Level

If you are just starting on your Keto Diet, it's best to restrict your carb intake to 20-30 grams per day (remember 1 big orange = 1 pint of beer = 20 grams carb). For a majority of people, carb intake range can be increased to 20-50 grams per day once you have achieved the desired weight loss and are in the weight maintenance phase. There are a number of Keto Calculator Apps you can find that will help you in calculating your exact macro proportions.

Mistake 2: Scale Watching

You need to accept the fact that being on a Keto Diet is a lifestyle change and not a crash diet. You will get there, keep calm and carry on!

It's natural for you to want to weigh yourself regularly to check progress when on a diet, but this is actually not a very accurate way to measure results. You need to realize that weight is just a number and is neither a very meaningful or accurate measure of how you are progressing nor an indicator of fat loss or physical fitness. Just remember that apart from your water weight that can fluctuate several pounds in a short span, the scale is a snapshot of what happened two weeks back.

What is the difference between your friend who weighs 300 lb. and an athlete who weighs the same? They do weigh the same but is their body composition the same?

It is important to understand that losing fat and weight are two different things. As we lose body fat and gain muscle mass especially for someone who has recently begun exercising, the scale would continue to show the same weight. Indicators that you are on track to losing weight even if the scale doesn't budge:

- Your tape measurements show a shrinking waistline.
- Your clothes are getting looser, you look slimmer and people around you notice the difference.
- You have lots of energy and want to exercise after living a sedentary lifestyle for years.
- Your health markers are improving.
- Your Body Mass Index (BMI) dips.
- Your mental focus improves, you don't experience afternoon slumps anymore.

Measure your Ketones

Measuring ketones is a good way to know that your body is in Ketosis and is burning the stored fat. There are a number of ways to measure ketones produced in your liver as your body goes through ketosis. These include urine test kits, blood test kits, breathalyzers and good old-fashioned observation techniques. Depending on your budget and interest, measuring ketones can be a good way to monitor results during ketogenic diet.

Mistake 3: Sugar Addiction

Sugar is the biggest hindrance to leading a healthy lifestyle. Removing sugar completely from your diet is absolutely necessary for a successful transition to Ketogenic Diet lifestyle. In fact, a gradual removal of this single substance from your diet alone will make you healthier than the majority of people. If you want to take one lesson from this book it is to completely remove sugar from your life.

The average per capita sugar consumption in America has risen to 153 grams per day from 9 grams per day back in 1822. Our bodies have got so used to sugar that in reality, it is difficult to get through a day without consuming sugar in some form. Being so readily available and ingrained in our lifestyle makes it all the more difficult to give up sweet foods. Check out the Resources section of the book for 56 different names of sugar used by the processed food industry to hide the amounts of added sugar in your food.

So what is Sugar? Sugar is simply Glucose + Fructose (The Sweet Part). It has:

- No healthy fats
- No protein
- No vitamins
- No enzymes

How Sugar makes us Eat More - Sugar triggers a chain reaction where high levels of sugar in the bloodstream results in increased insulin levels. This insulin, in turn, makes it difficult for the brain to receive the satiety signal. As a result, the brain is fooled to believe that the body is still hungry leading to excessive food consumption and weight gain.

How to Overcome Sugar Cravings:

- Reduce your Carb Intake: A high carb diet causes blood sugar to rise, which in turn signals the body to release insulin. You need to increase your consumption of protein and good fat to overcome this. Proteins are made up of amino acids, which are important for balancing hormones and sugar cravings. Healthy fats are a source of energy for our body and help reduce hunger pangs and provide satiety.

- Plan Your Meals in Advance: Hunger is not the best time to make rational decisions on what is best to eat. Planning ahead to include nutrient-rich food in your diet will help curb hunger swings and sugar cravings.
- L-Glutamine Dr. Julia Ross in her book "The Mood Curse" suggests that intense sugar cravings are due to stress, poor diet and deficiency of amino acids (to the extent that diet alone may not be able to correct it). She suggests a short-term supplementation of amino acid L- Glutamine.
- Check your Pantry: Keep sugary foods out of sight as much as possible.
- Watch Out for the Hidden Sugar: Low fat, sugar-free and diet foods contain added sugar or synthetic sweeteners in order to enhance the taste of the food and palatability. Get into the habit of going through the labeling for savory foods, juices, sauces, salad dressings and condiments. You will be surprised how many of them contain sugar.
- Avoid Artificial Sweeteners: Replacing sugar with a sugar substitute in the belief that it will reduce calorie intake and help in weight loss is a myth. Recent studies have shown that on the contrary artificial sweeteners

87

maintain the cravings for sweet food and increase appetite. Our body increases insulin secretion in anticipation that sugar will appear in the bloodstream. When the body doesn't receive the sugar, insulin uses the existing sugar in the bloodstream for energy. As a result, blood sugar levels drop and hunger increases leading to uncontrolled binging.

Mistake 4: Electrolyte Imbalance

Electrolytes are salts that flow in your bloodstream and carry an electric charge. They are essential for the cells in our body to function properly, whether it is to regulate blood pressure, help with muscle contraction or nervous system functions.

It is a well-known fact that on a Keto Diet the initial transition phase results in significant water loss. With the water are lost essential minerals like sodium and potassium, which triggers an electrolyte imbalance.

You will need about three times more electrolytes when on a Keto Diet as compared to a normal diet. Signs that you have an Electrolyte Imbalance:

- You are restless, have muscle aches, spasms and joint pains
- You have heart palpitations and find it difficult to sleep.
- You experience dizziness and fatigue I

Important Electrolytes Include:

Sodium

Responsible for maintaining fluid balance in our bodies, helps in muscle contraction and nerve signaling.

Sources of Sodium: Table Salt and Himalayan Pink Salt.

Magnesium:

One of the most under-appreciated minerals, Magnesium helps in maintaining a stable heart rate, bone building, the creation of DNA and RNA and normal nerve and muscle functions.

Sources of Magnesium: Almond, Salmon, Spices and Leafy Vegetables.

Potassium:

It aids muscle contraction, regulates heart contractions and keeps blood pressure stable. An imbalance of sodium and potassium is caused when we consume sodium-loaded processed foods and skip vegetables rich in potassium. This could lead to hypertension, heart attack and stroke.
Sources of Potassium: Avocado, Nuts and Dark Leafy Vegetables.

Calcium:

In addition to helping with the formation and maintenance of bones and teeth, calcium helps with cell division, cell clotting and transmission of nerve impulses.

Sources of Calcium: Almonds, Cheese and Broccoli.

Healthy individuals who are not working out extensively get their daily intake of electrolytes from the food they eat.

However, if you are sick, out on a very hot day or on a low carb diet, your electrolyte requirement spikes up.

Mistake 5: Fat Phobia

For years we have been told that eating fat will make you fat. Some of the most popular diets in the world are based on this premise. It is this social conditioning that leads us to subconsciously make choices that are low in fat.

As a result sugar and grains have been the primary source of the calories for most of us. Once you remove these two from your diet you will need to replace them with another energy source. If you don't you will feel hungry, tired and low all the time and will eventually switch back to carbs.

It is important to understand that there are two sources of energy – glucose and ketones. When on a low carb diet, sufficient intake of fat (60-75 % of total intake) leads us into ketosis and our body uses ketones for energy. However, if our body does not get into ketosis, it will look out for glucose for energy. It will either get it from carbohydrates or from protein (through Gluconeogenesis).

Keto Diet advocates a mix of saturated fats, omega 3s and monounsaturated fats.

Different types of Fat Present in our Food:

Saturated Fat (SFA):

They are stable fats, with long shelf life and suitable for high flame cooking. They help to keep in check your bone density, immune system and testosterone levels. Contrary to popular belief their consumption does not adversely affect the heart.

Sources of SFA: Meat, Egg, Butter, Ghee, Lard, Coconut Oil are good sources of Saturated Fat.

Monounsaturated Fat (MUFA):

They are liquid at room temperature and best for cold use for salads or after cooking. Good for the heart, they are now a popular choice of fat.

Sources of MUFA: Avocado, Olives and Nuts (especially macadamia).

Polyunsaturated Fat (PUFA):

This type of fats can be primarily divided into the naturally occurring Omega 3s and the industrially processed Omega 6 fats. PUFAs are unstable and fragile and not suitable for cooking. When heated, they react with oxygen to form harmful compounds called free radicals, which in turn raise our risk of heart diseases and cancer. Omega 3 consumption is good for our body but most of the PUFA cooking oil is high in omega 6, which is harmful.

The ideal ratio of Omega 6 to Omega 3 fats is 1: 1. However, in reality, the ratio is way higher than this, ranging from 10: 1 to 20: 1 on an average, so not only do we have a problem of excess Polyunsaturated fat, we also have a much higher proportion of omega 6 fats and deficiency of omega 3s.

Sources of healthy Omega 3s: Wild Salmon, Walnut, Fermented Cod Liver Oil, Macadamia Nuts and Grass-Fed Meat.

<u>Trans Fat:</u>

This is considered the worst form of fat and should be avoided. Trans fat is unsaturated fats primarily found in processed foods where through industrial process hydrogen is added to liquid vegetable oil to cause the fat to become solid at room temperature. This partially hydrogenated oil helps to increase the shelf life of processed food. It is linked to heart diseases and has an adverse effect on cholesterol levels.

Stay clear of products whose product label mentions words like "trans fat", "hydrogenated". It is worth noting that in the United States if per serving of any product anything lower than 0.5 grams then it can be labeled as 0 grams of trans fat. These hidden trans fats quickly add up if you consume multiple servings.

High-Fat Foods to Include in Your Diet:

- Avocados: Avocado, unlike most fruit, is loaded with monounsaturated fat oleic acid. This is the main fatty acid in olive oil and linked with various health benefits. It is a great source of potassium and fiber and helps lower triglyceride.
- Cheese: It is made from the milk of grass-fed animals is a good source of nutrients as it is high in saturated fats and omega 3-s, protein and amino acids
- Whole Eggs: Eggs are one of the most nutrient-dense foods and are loaded with vitamins and minerals.
- Fatty cuts of Meats and Fish: Include fatty cuts of grass-fed animals. Avoid chicken breasts or lean meat where the fat has been removed. Include fish like Salmon, Sardine, Mackerel and Trout in the meal plans. If you cannot eat fish then it is worth considering a supplement like Cod fish liver oil, which contains Omega 3-s and Vitamin D.

- Nuts: Nuts are loaded with Protein, Vitamin E and Magnesium in addition to healthy fats and are a great option to add to a meal when consumed in moderation. Almonds, Walnuts and Macadamia nuts are some of the healthy choices.
- Chia seeds: They are high in Omega 3 fatty acids and fiber. They can be a useful addition to your diet.
- Extra Virgin Olive Oil: Rich in vitamin E & K and loaded with antioxidants, extra virgin Olive oil is an excellent choice. The antioxidants in the oil help improve cardiovascular health, lower blood pressure, fight inflammation and protect LDL particles from oxidation in the blood.
- Coconut Oil: It contains 90% saturated fatty acids making it the richest source of saturated fat.
- Butter and Ghee (clarified butter): Butter has been demonized for long but Grass Fed butter is good for you. In addition to Vitamin A, E and K2 it contains Conjugated Linoleic Acid (CLA) and Butyrate. CLA helps in lowering fat percentage and Butyrate improves the gut and fights inflammation.
- Lard, Tallow and Bacon Fat from naturally raised animals are a great option for cooking and are high in healthy saturated and monounsaturated fats

Mistake 6: Carb-Loaded

So much has already been discussed about carbs. But I would like to reiterate that you should become aware of your carb tolerance. An athlete will probably have a greater carb tolerance than someone with a sedentary lifestyle. On the safer side, your carbs intake should not go beyond 20 grams max when you start your Keto Diet.

Getting rid of carbs may work in the short term, but there always comes a time when all of us start to crave for the starchy stuff. The temptation of having just that one small slice of bread can be overwhelming.

Let me warn you again though, Ketosis is a reversible state and can be broken very easily by just having that one small piece. Not only that, once you start eating that one piece, insulin level in your blood starts to rise which will play all kinds of havoc with you. Let me show you how a high carb diet affects us physiologically.

Why "Eat less and Exercise more" is Not a Solution: The conventional weight loss wisdom from the diet industry is 'Eat less and Exercise more'. This advice, derived from the calorie in calorie out (CICO) theory, falls flat in the world of complex human physiology. CICO completely ignores the inner workings of a human body and has led to lots of people abandoning their weight loss quest.

People who propagate CICO believe that Calorie IN = Calorie OUT + Stored Fat. So the amount of fat stored in the body depends upon the number of calories we consume minus the calories expended in bodily functions and exercise. Nothing can be far from the truth!

The human body has no way of measuring calories but has its own way of regulating fat. Insulin is the hormone that controls how much energy we expend and how much is stored as fat.

When we eat, the insulin goes up and the body starts storing fat. And eating equal calories of carb will raise insulin level more that eating equal calories of fat. That's why in human physiology; a calorie is not a calorie. As we stop eating, the insulin levels drop and the body stops storing fat. As the fasting continues body starts burning the stored fat.

That's why conventional (High Carb Low Fat) diets fail. Because of high insulin levels in carb-based diets, fat is being continuously stored. So even if you are eating lesser calories overall, insulin levels will remain high because of carb consumption and fat storage will continue. Ironically, weight gain continues and with increased appetite.

In a Low Carb High Fat (LCHF) diet, however, the insulin levels are lower. So when you consume equal calories of fat based food, a part of your energy needs will be met with the stored body fat. So using an LCHF diet for fat loss is more effective as your appetite is decreasing with a steady decline in body fat.

Mistake 7: Excessive Drinking

Keto Diet does not mean the end of your social life. Sure hit the bars, but you have to do so responsibly. Please remember if it tastes sweet, it's probably sugary and should be avoided.

You will have to keep a check on what you drink and how much you drink. Beer and wine should be especially avoided as they contain a lot of carbs and sugar. When you drink, your body will metabolize it on priority before other sources of energy, as it cannot store alcohol. This means that although alcohol consumption will not completely throw you out of ketosis it will for sure prolong the timeline for your goals as when the body is burning alcohol for energy it is unable to metabolize the stored fat.

Remember to drink plenty of water in between your drinks. Keto lowers your alcohol tolerance level so keep sufficient gap between drinks.

Mistake 8: Importance of Proteins

Like many of us do you also have the notion that Ketogenic Diet is all about keeping your carbs low and increasing your fat intake?

For a lot of people just keeping low on carbs, helps in weight loss. However, some people are more metabolically resistant than others and despite keeping their carb levels below 20 grams per day continue to gain weight. It is in such cases worth looking at your protein intake.

We give little attention to how much protein we need to consume in order to stay in ketosis. Our body cannot make protein on its own and as such protein is an important macronutrient without which your body wouldn't be able to carry out the necessary tissue building and repair functions.

What is Gluconeogenesis?

It is worth understanding the process of gluconeogenesis here. It is a metabolic process by which our body produces glucose from non-carbohydrate sources – amino acids in the protein being one of them.

Gluconeogenesis is an essential process without which we probably cannot survive for long, especially if we need to go without food, as our body needs a constant and steady flow of glucose to keep the brain and red blood cells functioning.

When we consume more protein than our body needs the excess is turned into glucose. This glucose is over and above the minimum requirement of the body and results in weight gain.

Optimum Protein Intake:

There are various theories on how you can calculate the ideal protein intake taking your weight in pounds and then multiply it by 0.6 and 1.0. This will then give you the ideal range for your protein intake in grams.

An easier way is to pick a level of protein and while still keeping carbs below 20 grams monitor how you are doing for that quantity of protein intake. If you continue to struggle, keep shifting your intake downwards until you hit the sweet spot.

It is worth noting that when you are experimenting to find your ideal level of protein intake you must keep your carbs low and have adequate monounsaturated and saturated fats to give you the much-needed satiety.

If you are struggling with weight loss due to being more sensitive to proteins, try and avoid leaner cuts of meat like chicken breast as that would elevate your blood sugar levels and make you gain weight just by having too much protein than your body needs. On the other side, cuts of meats with saturated fat will automatically lower your protein intake and help in weight loss.

Mistake 9: Falling for Fake Products

Wouldn't it be great if we could eat bread, pasta and chocolate and still lose weight rapidly without hunger or all the complicated diseases associated with sugar?

There are plenty of shady businesses that promise the impossible. An excellent example is low carb pasta from Dreamfields that tastes like any regular pasta. They are even made from regular starchy wheat, but the manufacturer still claims that our body does not absorb the carbs as their pasta is protected from some "patent pending process".

The problem is that their claims are completely bogus and raises blood sugar like any regular pasta. Based on several types of research it was proved that their pasta behaved like regular pasta and Dreamfields had to pay a settlement fine of $ 8 million because they had lied; however, by then they had sold their fake low carb pasta for 10 years.

There are many similar examples of fake products. Carbzone is a company that claims to sell low carb products. They claim their tortilla made from whole wheat is low carb; however, on testing it showed to contain 3 times as many carbs as stated on the label. Even low carb chocolate cookies from the Atkins Company often contain sugar alcohol like Maltitol, which the maker pretends to not raise blood sugar. However, this claim has no merit and about half of it does end up raising blood sugar. The manufactures omit sugar alcohols from the net carb count so that they can market it as low carb.

In short, do not fall for fake products. If it tastes like bread, pasta or chocolate then the reality is that it is bread, pasta and chocolate.

Lifestyle Problems

Now, let's look at the lifestyle challenges that some followers may face. We will also look at the best ways that these can be addressed.

Keto on a Budget

Some people worry about following Ketogenic Diet on a budget. But actually, once you start, you'll find that your monthly spend on food will actually go down. The reasons for the same are mentioned below:
1. You will buy fresh base ingredients instead of processed ingredients
2. Once you hit ketosis, you will observe that satiety comes much earlier and you will eat less. This is another sign that you are in the state of Ketosis.

Farmer's market is a great place to shop for fresh ingredients while on Keto. You will find pocket-friendly bargains

there while supporting the local community. Moreover, you will learn more about your food by being in direct touch with the producers.

Eating Out

Eating in a restaurant can seem daunting when you first start following a ketogenic diet. Actually, it doesn't need to be difficult if you follow a few simple rules.

Try to stick to meat, dairy, or vegetable dishes that don't come with rice, pasta, or bread. Things like steak with salad are a good choice, as are salads on their own with cheese or meat added. Other good choices when eating out can be fish or seafood with non-starchy vegetables.

Just be careful to have them with olive oil rather than dressings, which can be high in sugar. Also remember that it is up to you if you want to customize your order and ask for things like sauces to be left out, so don't be afraid to ask! It also is worth checking with the restaurants if they have Keto/ Paleo/ LCHF friendly dishes.

Eating with Friends and Family

Friends and family may not understand Ketogenic Diet and may want you to eat whatever they are eating, especially if you have done so in the past. At the end of the day, you may not be able to explain the principles of Ketogenic Diet to them in a way that changes their minds, but just remember that it is up to you to choose what to eat. They may just be convinced when they see your weight loss and renewed energy levels!

Conclusion

The keto diet can be hard to maintain which is why you should try to get into it slowly. The first step is to slowly transition yourself into it instead of just pushing your body to the limit. So, don't abandon all the food that you used to eat, instead cut them out of your diet slowly.

The second step is to jump right into it and wait for the benefits to start showing. Now, it might happen that the diet isn't working for you, but you shouldn't worry about that. Our bodies are different which is why not all diets can work for everyone. You should consult your doctor if you are not losing any weight even after following the diet for a long time.

Lastly, remember to stay motivated and tell yourself why you're doing this. It can be hard to cut out all the carbs from your life, but you can always use some simple techniques to keep yourself motived. You should take pictures of yourself after every few months and notice the progress you are making, this will help you to stay on track.

Finally, if you enjoyed this book, then I'd like to ask you for a favor, would you be kind enough to leave a review for this book on Amazon? It'd be greatly appreciated!

Thank you and good luck!

Preview Of Intermittent fasting:
**Beginners Guide To Weight Loss For Men
And Women With Intermittent Fasting**

Do you want a diet that will help you lose weight and improve your overall health? Do you want a diet that doesn't prescribe calorie counting? It does sound quite wonderful if you can achieve your weight loss and health goals without counting calories, doesn't it? If your answer is yes, then you are in for a pleasant surprise! Intermittent Fasting is the diet that you have been looking for. Fasting is not a new concept and has been around for a long time. Intermittent Fasting is a simple variation of fasting and is very helpful. This dieting protocol alternates between periods of fasting and eating.

In this book, you will learn about the basics of Intermittent Fasting, the changes that take place in your body, the benefits it offers, different methods of Intermittent Fasting, tips to exercise, common FAQs and much more. Intermittent Fasting is quite simple. You merely need to make a couple of changes to your eating habits and you are good to go.

If you are fascinated by this diet and want to learn more about it, then let us start right now!

Chapter One:
History of Intermittent Fasting

U nlike other forms of conventional dieting, the concept of fasting is quite unambiguous and easy to understand. Did you know that most of us tend to unconsciously follow the protocols of Intermittent Fasting? Do you ever skip having breakfast or dinner? If you do, then you are following an Intermittent Fasting protocol. You will learn about the different methods of Intermittent Fasting in the coming chapters.

Our hunter and gatherer caveman ancestors had to seek food in nature. So, they were often on a fast until they found some nourishment. Then agriculture was introduced, and it led to the formation of human civilization. Whenever there was food scarcity or whenever the seasons changed, fasting was the norm. They used to maintain stocks of grain and meat in cities and castles for harsh winters. Before the introduction of agriculture, shortage of rainfall meant a spell of famine and people used to fast to make their food supplies last longer. Enough rain was quintessential to meet the grain requirement.

Along with civilizations, there came religions. Religions grew when people were living in close quarters and shared similar beliefs. Most of the religions prescribe fasting. Hinduism refers to fasting as Vaasa, and Hindus observe it during festivals or other auspicious days. Fasting is also considered to be a form of penance. Islam prescribes fasting during the holy month of Ramzan. A similar practice is present in Judaism and is known as Yom Kippur. There's a period of fasting before Easter in the Catholic faith.

Technology and innovations play a vital role in the evolution of humans. Industrialization revolutionized the food industry. Mass production of food products meant that the markets were constantly flooded with food products. Apart from this, the way humans view and consume food has also undergone a major change. The human body didn't get a chance to sufficiently adapt itself to the rampant changes brought about by industrialization and agriculture. All this meant that a host of health problems soon followed. Intermittent Fasting is quite an old practice. Even though it is an old practice, humans have just begun to understand and truly appreciate the various benefits this diet offers. Whenever you fast, you give your body a chance to cleanse itself - not just cleanse but even repair and regenerate itself from within.

Essentially, while fasting your body gets to burn out all the excess fat it has stored. Human beings have evolved in such a manner that we can fast without any health risks and that is normal. Body fat is the reserve of food that the body has stashed away for a rainy day. If you don't consume food, your body will simply reach into this reserve to provide you with energy. There needs to be balance in everything you do. There's a yin and a yang. The same rule applies to eating and fasting as well. Fasting is the flip side of eating. If you aren't eating, then you are fasting. When you eat something, this leads to an accumulation of food energy that isn't going to be made use of immediately. A portion of this is stored away. A hormone known as insulin is responsible for storing the food energy. When you eat something, there is a spike in the level of insulin. This facilitates the storage of energy in two different ways. Sugars are linked into long chains and this is known as glycogen. The rest is stored in the liver. When the space available has been maxed out, the liver starts turning the rest into fat. Some of this fat so created is stored in the liver and the rest is stored in the form of fat cells in the rest of your body. There isn't a limit on fat creation. So, there are two forms of energy stores in our bodies. One is easily accessible and has a limited storage space (glycogen), and the other is the harder to reach energy without a limit on storage (body fat).

This process is essentially reversed when you don't eat, that is during fasting. There will be a reduction in the level of insulin and this enables your body to reach into its storage of fat cells and burn this to provide energy. The most easily attainable source of energy for your body is glycogen. This is broken down into molecules of glucose that sustains your body. This can provide sufficient energy for your body to function for 24 hours or longer. After this, your body will reach into its fat reserves to generate energy. Your body will do this only while feeding or fasting. Either your body will be storing energy, or it will be burning energy. Only either of these processes can take place at any given time. If there is a balance between eating and fasting, then there will not be any weight gain. Over a period of time, you will start gaining weight if you haven't given your body sufficient time to burn all the food it has stored. To restore balance, you will need to give your body sufficient time to burn the food energy. This can be accomplished by fasting. This is how our bodies are designed. Intermittent Fasting helps to restore this much-needed balance.

Circadian Rhythm and Intermittent Fasting

Human beings, like other organisms, have a biological circadian clock that ensures that the physiological processes in the body are performed at the right time. The circadian rhythm is on all day long and it affects the biology and the behavior of humans. Any disruption in this rhythm has a negative effect on the metabolism and it can cause several metabolic dysfunctions like obesity, diabetes and a host of cardiovascular diseases. The primary factor that affects the circadian rhythm is the signal to eat. It is responsible for metabolic, physiological and behavioral pathways in the body. All these pathways are responsible for making sure that your body performs optimally. Apart from this, they also ensure that your body is healthy. You can use behavioral intervention to regulate the body's circadian rhythm. Yes, you guessed it right! Intermittent Fasting is a means of behavioral intervention that will streamline the circadian rhythm. This in turn leads to better gene expression and improvement in your body's health and metabolism.

Gut Microbiome and Intermittent Fasting

The gastrointestinal tract regulates multiple processes within your body. In other words, your gut helps regulate different physiological and biochemical functions in your body. For instance, the metabolic reaction to glucose and the blood flow are higher during the day than at night. Even a small fluctuation in the circadian rhythm can impair your metabolism and increases the risk of several chronic diseases. The microbiome present in the gut is usually referred to as the second brain. It is known as the second brain because of the influence it has over your metabolism and physiology. Intermittent Fasting has a positive impact on the gut microbiome. It makes the gut less permeable, reduces the chances of systemic inflammation and improves overall energy balance.

Lifestyle Behavior and Intermittent Fasting

Intermittent Fasting helps change different health-related behaviors like calorie consumption, energy expenditure and your sleep cycle. Therefore, it is not a surprise that these are the three primary functions that help fight the most significant health concern that plagues the human community, obesity. You will learn more about the different benefits it offers in the coming chapters.

Chapter Two:
Different Methods of Fasting

I ntermittent Fasting is a varied and a dynamic diet that offers multiple health benefits. There are different methods of Intermittent Fasting that you can follow, and you need to select one that will meet your needs. So, read on to learn more about the different methods of Intermittent Fasting.

16/8 Method

If you follow this method of Intermittent Fasting, you must fast for 16 hours daily. If you fast for 16 hours, the eating window comes down to 8 hours. You can squeeze in two or three healthy meals within this time frame. It is popularly known as the LeanGains method. The creator of this variant of Intermittent Fasting was Martin Berkhan, a fitness expert. This method can be something as simple as skipping your breakfast and directly having your first meal at noon and your last one at about 8 p.m.

The next meal you can have will be on the following day at noon. So, you will fast for 16 hours and, frankly, you will not even feel like you were fasting for 16 hours. Ideally, women must not fast for more than 14 hours. If you like to wake up early and eat breakfast, then have a hearty breakfast, then you need to make sure that your last meal is at around 4 or 6 in the evening.

You are free to consume all sorts of calorie-free beverages throughout the day like water, black coffee or any other herbal teas. You need to make sure that you don't include any sugar in your drinks, since it will effectively break your fast. If you want to lose weight, then you must not binge on junk foods when you break your fast. This method works, only if you strictly follow the protocols of the diet.

The 5:2 Diet

In this variation of the diet, you need to restrict your calorie intake on two days of the week and eat like you normally do on the other days. On the days you need to restrict your calorie intake, the calories you consume must be between 500 and 600. Michael Mosley is the creator of this diet and it is also known as the Fast diet. On the days that you fast, you must ensure you don't consume more than 600 calories. You can squeeze in two small meals within this calorie limit. This diet is ideal for all those who don't like the idea of fasting daily.

Eat-stop-Eat

In this form of Intermittent Fasting, you must fast for 24 hours, once or twice in a week. Brad Pilon, a famous fitness expert, created this diet.

You can choose the days you want to fast on. For instance, if your fast starts at 8 p.m. on Monday night, then you will break your fast only at 8 p.m. on Tuesday night. You can decide when you want to fast, if you fast for 24-hours. You cannot consume any solid food during your fasting period but can have calorie-free beverages. You must ensure that you are consuming healthy meals on the normal days. If you are just getting started with fasting, then this might be a little complicated. Instead, it is a good idea to start with either of the previous methods and then make your way toward this dieting protocol. If you want to follow this diet, then you need self-discipline and self-control.

Make sure that your fasting period never exceeds 48 hours. So, don't try to fast on two days continuously and pace it evenly.

Alternate Day Fasting

If you want to follow this method of Intermittent Fasting, then you need to consume 500 calories on every alternate day. If you are not a fan of a strict diet, then this will work well for you. You can eat like you normally do on all days except for the ones with the calorie restriction.

Warrior Diet

Ori Hofmekler, a famous fitness expert, was the creator of this diet. In this method, you need to have small portions of raw fruits and vegetables during the day and end your day with a hearty meal at night. You will essentially be fasting throughout the day and will feast at night. The eating window in this method is restricted to about 4 hours. The food that you can consume on this diet is quite like the food you can consume while following a Paleo diet. So, you are free to fill up on foods that are unprocessed. It essentially means that you can eat only those foods that our cavemen ancestors had access to. If you feel like your caveman ancestors could not have eaten something, then neither can you. If you don't want to fast all day long, you can snack on fruit and vegetables. It will keep your hunger pangs at bay.

Spontaneous Fasting

As the name suggests, you merely need to skip meals spontaneously. There is no fixed plan. If you don't feel like eating, you simply need to skip a meal. There will be times when you don't have time to eat or when you don't feel like eating. So, whenever you skip a meal, you are effectively following the protocols of this diet. It will not do your body any harm if you skip meals from time to time.

Chapter Three:
Benefits of Intermittent Fasting

Perhaps the most common reason why people opt for Intermittent Fasting is to lose weight. Apart from weight loss, there are various other benefits this diet offers, and you will learn about them in this chapter.

Weight loss

Intermittent Fasting alternates between periods of eating and fasting. If you fast, naturally your calorie intake will reduce, and it also helps you maintain your weight loss. It also prevents you from indulging in mindless eating. Whenever you eat something, your body converts the food into glucose and fat. It uses the glucose immediately and stores the fat for later use. When you skip a few meals, your body starts to reach into its internal stores of fat to provide energy. As soon as your body starts burning fats due to the shortage of glucose, you will start to lose weight. Also, most of the fat that you lose is from the abdominal region. If you want a flat tummy, then this is the perfect diet for you.

Sleep

Lack of sleep is a primary cause of obesity. When your body doesn't get enough sleep, the internal mechanism of burning fat suffers. Intermittent Fasting regulates your sleep cycle and, in turn, it makes your body effectively burn fats. A good sleep cycle has different physiological benefits - it makes you feel energetic and elevates your overall mood.

Resistance to illnesses

Intermittent Fasting helps in the growth and the regeneration of cells. Did you know that the human body has an internal mechanism that helps repair damaged cells? Intermittent Fasting helps kickstart this mechanism. It improves the overall functioning of all the cells in the body. So, it is directly responsible for improving your body's natural defense mechanism by increasing its resistance to diseases and illnesses.

A healthy heart

Intermittent Fasting assists in weight loss, and weight loss improves your cardiovascular health. A buildup of plaque in blood vessels is known as atherosclerosis. This is the primary cause for various cardiovascular diseases. Endothelium is the thin lining of blood vessels and any dysfunction in it results in atherosclerosis. Obesity is the primary problem that plagues humanity and is also the main reason for the increase of plaque deposits in the blood vessels. Stress and inflammation also increase the severity of this problem. Intermittent Fasting tackles the buildup of fat and helps tackle obesity. So, all you need to do is follow the simple protocols of Intermittent Fasting to improve your overall health.

A healthy gut

There are several millions of microorganisms present in your digestive system. These microorganisms help improve the overall functioning of your digestive system and are known as gut microbiome. Intermittent

Fasting improves the health of these microbiome and improves your digestive health. A healthy digestive system helps in better absorption of food and improves the functioning of your stomach.

Tackles diabetes

Diabetes is a serious problem on its own. It is also a primary indicator of the increase in risk factors of various cardiovascular diseases like heart attacks and strokes. When the glucose level increases alarmingly in the bloodstream and there isn't enough insulin to process this glucose, it causes diabetes. When the body is resistant to insulin, it becomes difficult to regulate the insulin levels in the body. Intermittent Fasting reduces insulin sensitivity and helps tackle diabetes.

Reduces inflammation

Whenever your body feels there is an internal problem, its natural defense is inflammation. It doesn't mean that all forms of inflammation are desirable. Inflammation can cause several serious health conditions like arthritis, atherosclerosis and other neurodegenerative disorders.

Any inflammation of this nature is known as chronic inflammation and is quite painful. Chronic inflammation can restrict your body's movements too. If you want to keep inflammation in check, then Intermittent Fasting will certainly come in handy.

Promotes cell repair

When you fast, the cells in your body start the process of waste removal. Waste removal means the breaking down of all dysfunctional cells and proteins and is known as autophagy. Autophagy offers protection against several degenerative diseases like Alzheimer's and cancer. You don't like accumulating garbage in your home, do you?

Similarly, your body must not hold onto any unnecessary toxins. Autophagy is the body's way of getting rid of all things unnecessary.

Chapter Four:
What to Avoid During a Fast

Intermittent Fasting helps rectify and reverse several health conditions, but it doesn't mean that it is ideal for everyone. An important thing that you need to keep in mind is that you need to consult your medical practitioner before you start this diet.

Who can fast?

The following people can fast

Healthy adults

All healthy adults can fast. It helps cleanse the body and there aren't any reasons why a healthy adult cannot fast.

Children

Usually, it isn't suitable for children up to the age of 18 to fast; however, children can fast. A child must only fast for a short duration and must not fast for prolonged periods. A perfectly healthy child doesn't have to fast. The general exception to this rule is all those who suffer from obesity. A child needs plenty of nutrition for growth and their body needs nourishment constantly. If the child is less than 18 years, please consult a medical practitioner.

Type-2 diabetes

Fasting helps reverse the harmful effects of type-2 diabetes. If you suffer from this, then you are free to fast. Before you start any diet, you must always consult your medical practitioner.

Who Cannot Fast?

Pregnant women

As such, there is no conclusive proof that shows the effect of Intermittent Fasting on a fetus. It is better to abstain from any diets if you are pregnant or are trying to conceive. If you are planning to start a family, then your body needs plenty of nutrition and you must not restrict your diet at this point of time. Also, mothers who are breast-feeding need to abstain from Intermittent Fasting. Fasting reduces the nutrition available in breast milk and it also affects the quantity of milk that is produced.

Any medical conditions

If you have any health concerns related to the kidney or the liver, then you must not fast. You need to consult a doctor before you fast if you have any pre-existing medical conditions. If you use any medication for high blood pressure or have a weak immune system, then you must not fast. You can fast even if you have medical conditions, but don't forget to consult your doctor.

If you have recently had a major surgery, then please abstain from fasting. Also, fasting is not ideal for all those who are recovering from any major illness.

Eating disorders

If you have any eating disorders or are recovering from an eating disorder, then you must not fast. Fasting can cause a relapse and you need to avoid it at any cost.

Afraid to fast

If fasting scares you, then don't fast. Fear is an unnecessary stressor and it will just cause problems. Fear is a powerful emotion and can alter your psychological makeup. If you think you cannot handle fasting, then don't try to fast. If you want this diet to generate positive results, you need to have an open mindset!

Foods to Avoid and Eat

When you are following the protocols of Intermittent Fasting, the primary focus is not on what you eat, but it is on when you eat. Just because it doesn't focus on what you eat, it doesn't mean that you stuff yourself with carbs and sugar-laden treats. For best results, it is a good idea to stay away from all processed foods and opt for healthy foods. It means that it is a good idea to avoid all sugary treats or at least try to limit them as much as you possibly can. So, avoid cookies, chocolates, cakes, and all packaged sweets.

Stay away from foods rich in unhealthy fats and carbs like burgers, pizzas and all fast foods. Say no to foods that are devoid of all protein and are full of sugars and carbs. Avoid soy products if you want to lose weight. Soy products are rich in estrogen and a high level of estrogen will not do you any good.

You need to maintain a calorie deficit if you want to lose weight. The higher the level of insulin in your body, the less fat you will lose. Carbs and sugars increase the level of insulin. So, if you want to regulate your insulin levels, you need to avoid carbs.

There are some people who believe that you can eat a lot of protein, fruit and vegetables while fasting. If you eat all this during a fast, you aren't effectively fasting, are you? Even if you had a couple of drops of honey to your morning tea, you will be effectively breaking your fast. Just because you aren't permitted to eat anything, doesn't mean that you stop drinking water.

Your body needs at least 8 glasses of water to stay hydrated and ensure that you are thoroughly hydrated. Drinking water will make you feel fuller and helps you to avoid any hunger pangs.

You are free to consume all calorie-free beverages like black tea, black coffee, green tea, herbal teas and carbonated water. Try to limit your caffeine intake. Caffeine has a diuretic effect on the body and too much of it can cause dehydration due to the loss of electrolytes. Try to limit your caffeine intake to about two cups of coffee or any other caffeinated calorie-free drink of your choice. It might seem quite tempting to add some sugar or cream to your coffee, or perhaps some honey to your tea. If you do this, you will cause a spike in your insulin levels. When there is a spike in your insulin levels, your body stops burning fat and it negates the benefits of fasting. You must try to avoid anything that will cause a spike in your insulin levels and effectively break your fast. Some people believe that chewing sugar-free gum will keep hunger at bay. Even all those products that are labeled as "no sugar" or "sugar-free" include some carbs in them.

If you really want to lose weight and want to improve your overall health, then it is a good idea to stay away from all forms of alcoholic drinks as well.

Alcohol contains a lot of carbs that can sneak up on you unknowingly. Intermittent Fasting helps cleanse your body. So, if you really want to cleanse your body then you need to avoid all the things that will result in the internal buildup of toxins. So, stay away from alcohol to improve the efficiency of this diet.

Lean & Green

Table of Contents

Introduction 1

Chapter 1. Lean and Green Foods 4

Chapter 2. Breakfast Recipes 8

1. Sun-Dried Tomato Garlic Bruschetta 8

2. Gingerbread Oatmeal Breakfast 9

3. Oat Porridge With Cherry & Coconut 10

4. Hash Browns 11

5. Apple Ginger and Rhubarb Muffins 12

6. Anti-Inflammatory Breakfast Frittata 13

7. White and Green Quiche 14

8. Yummy Steak Muffins 15

9. Breakfast Sausage and Mushroom Casserole 16

10. Mushroom Crêpes 18

11. Beef Breakfast Casserole 20

12. Fantastic Spaghetti Squash With Cheese and Basil Pesto 21

13. Ham and Veggie Frittata Muffins 22

14. Cheesy Flax and Hemp Seeds Muffins 23

15. Cheddar and Chive Souffles 24

16. Shirataki Pasta With Avocado and Cream 25

17. Mango Granola 26

18. Blueberry & Cashew Waffles 27

19. Tomato and Avocado Omelet 28

20. Vegan-Friendly Banana Bread 29

Chapter 3. Side Dish Recipes 30

21. Plant-Powered Pancakes 30

22. Hemp Seed Porridge 31

23. Walnut Crunch Banana Bread 32

24. Mini Mac in a Bowl 33

25. Mini Zucchini Bites 34

26. Lean and Green Smoothie 2 35

27. Mushroom & Spinach Omelet 36

28. Whole-Wheat Blueberry Muffins 37

29. Sweet Cashew Cheese Spread 38

30. Mouthwatering Tuna Melts...39

31. Easiest Tuna Cobbler Ever 40

32. Lean and Green Smoothie 1 41

33. Deliciously Homemade Pork Buns..................................42

34. Yogurt Garlic Chicken 43

35. Tuna Spinach Casserole..45

36. Lean and Green Chicken Pesto Pasta............................46

37. Open-Face Egg Sandwiches With Cilantro-Jalapeño Spread 47

38. Lemony Parmesan Salmon...49

39. Chicken Omelet..50

40. Pepper Pesto Lamb 51

41. Best Whole Wheat Pancakes..52

42. Spiced Pumpkin Muffins...53

Chapter 4. Salads 54

43. Blueberry Cantaloupe Avocado Salad 54

44. Wild Rice Prawn Salad...55

45. Beet Salad (from Israel) 56

46. Greek Salad 57

47. Norwegian Niçoise Salad Smoked Salmon Cucumber Egg and
Asparagus 58

48. Mediterranean Chickpea Salad......................................59

49. Romaine Lettuce and Radicchios Mix.............................60

50. Chicken Broccoli Salad With Avocado Dressing.............61

51. Zucchini Salmon Salad 62

52. Warm Chorizo Chickpea Salad 63

53. Broccoli Salad 64

Chapter 5. Soup and Stew Recipes 65

54. Roasted Tomato Soup 65

55. Lemon-Garlic Chicken.. 66

56. Quick Lentil Chili 67

57. Creamy Cauliflower Soup 68

58. Crackpot Chicken Taco Soup 69

59. Cheeseburger Soup 70

60. Mushroom & Jalapeño Stew 71

61. Easy Cauliflower Soup 72

62. Tofu Stir Fry With Asparagus Stew 73

63. Cream of Thyme Tomato Soup.. 74

64. Lime-Mint Soup 75

Chapter 6. Vegan Recipes 76

65. Vegan Edamame Quinoa Collard Wraps.................................... 76

66. Baked Cheesy Eggplant With Marinara 78

67. Creamy Spinach and Mushroom Lasagna................................... 79

68. Zucchini Parmesan Chips 81

69. Roasted Squash Puree 82

70. Air Fryer Brussels Sprouts 83

71. Thai Roasted Veggies 84

72. Crispy Jalapeno Coins 85

73. Crispy-Topped Baked Vegetables 86

74. Jicama Fries 87

75. Spaghetti Squash Tots.. 88

76. Low Carb Pork Dumplings With Dipping Sauce........................... 89

77. Gluten-Free Air Fryer Chicken Fried Brown Rice 90

78. Air Fryer Cheesy Pork Chops 91

79. Air Fryer Pork Chop & Broccoli 92

80. Mustard Glazed Air Fryer Pork Tenderloin 93

81. Air Fryer Pork Taquitos 94

82. Pork Rind Nachos 95

83. Air Fried Jamaican Jerk Pork 96

84. Beef Lunch Meatballs 97

85. Air Fryer Whole Wheat Crusted Pork Chops 98

86. Air Fried Philly Cheesesteak Taquitos 99

Chapter 8. Snacks and Party Food 100

87. Salmon Sandwich With Avocado and Egg 100

88. Tasty Onion and Cauliflower Dip 101

89. Marinated Eggs 102

90. Pumpkin Muffins 103

91. Salmon Spinach and Cottage Cheese Sandwich 104

92. Sausage and Cheese Dip 105

93. Pesto Crackers 106

94. Bacon Cheeseburger 107

95. Cheeseburger Pie 108

96. Smoked Salmon and Cheese on Rye Bread 109

97. Chicken and Mushrooms 110

98. Chicken Enchilada Bake 111

99. Salmon Feta and Pesto Wrap 112

100. Pan-Fried Trout 113

101. Glazed Bananas in Phyllo Nut Cups 114

102. Salmon Cream Cheese and Onion on Bagel 115

103. Greek Baklava 117

104. Easy Salmon Burger 118

105. White Bean Dip 119

106. Grilled Salmon Burger 120

Chapter 9. Desserts Recipes 121

107. Chocolate Bars 121

108. Blueberry Muffins 122

109. Chocolate Fondue 123

110. Apple Crisp 124

111. Yogurt Mint 125

112. Raspberry Compote 126

113. Braised Apples 127

114. Rice Pudding 128

115. Rhubarb Dessert 129

116. Wine Figs 130

117. Chia Pudding 131

Chapter 10. Air Fryer Meals and Breakfast Recipes 132

118. Cloud Focaccia Bread Breakfast 132

119. Cloud Garlic Bread Breakfast 133

120. Cheesy Broccoli Bites 134

121. Portabella Mushrooms Stuffed With Cheese 135

122. Bell-Pepper Wrapped in Tortilla 136

123. Air Fried Cauliflower Ranch Chips 137

124. Brine & Spinach Egg Air Fried Muffins 138

125. Coconut Battered Cauliflower Bites 139

126. Crispy Roasted Broccoli 140

127. Crispy Cauliflowers 141

128. Red Pepper & Kale Air Fried Egg Muffins 142

Chapter 11. Side Dish Recipes 143

129. Low Carb Air-Fried Calzones 143

130. Air-Fried Tortilla Hawaiian Pizza 144

131. Tasty Kale & Celery Crackers 145

132. Air Fryer Personal Mini Pizza 146

133. Air Fried Cheesy Chicken Omelet 147

134. 5-Ingredients Air Fryer Lemon Chicken 148

135. Air Fryer Popcorn Chicken 149

136. Air Fryer Chicken Nuggets 150

137. Air Fryer Sweet & Sour Chicken 151

138. Low Carb Chicken Tenders.. 152

139. Cheesy Cauliflower Tots 153

Chapter 18. Dessert Recipes...154

140. Bread Dough and Amaretto Dessert 154

141. Bread Pudding.. 155

142. Wrapped Pears 156

143. Air Fried Bananas... 157

144. Tasty Banana Cake 158

145. Peanut Butter Fudge 159

146. Cocoa Cake.. 160

147. Avocado Pudding 161

148. Bounty Bars.. 162

149. Simple Cheesecake 163

150. Chocolate Almond Butter Brownie 164

151. Almond Butter Fudge 165

152. Apple Bread.. 166

153. Banana Bread 167

154. Mini Lava Cakes... 168

155. Ricotta Ramekins 169

156. Strawberry Sorbet 170

157. Crispy Apples 171

158. Cocoa Cookies 172

159. Cinnamon Pears... 173

160. Cherry Compote 174

Introduction

Lean and green diet is a special variant of the low-fat diet, which further makes use of lean proteins instead of fat in promoting weight loss and improving health. Lean protein sources include skinless poultry, fish (e.g. cod and haddock), lean cuts of meat, eggs and vegetable proteins such as lentils and beans. This kind of diet improves the metabolism by increasing the metabolic rate that speeds up weight loss. It also reduces the risk of obesity, because following the lean and green diet does not increase body fat as much as low-fat diets.

The emphasis is on consuming a small amount of meat and fish that are eaten twice a day, together with other protein sources such as eggs, lentils and beans. The diet includes vegetables in addition to fruits that are rich in vitamins (e.g. carrots). The green food includes different varieties of beans like green lentils, black-eyed peas and soybeans. Lean and Green diet is one of the healthy diets that should be consumed frequently, because it complements all other healthy diets.

Recent studies show that lean diets have similar results to low fat diets in reducing body weight. The lean and green diet, however, do not show a considerable improvement in the health risk factors like blood lipids, blood pressure and insulin resistance compared to low-fat diets.

A green lean and cleanse diet, or simply green lean diet, is a diet similar to the concept of a raw food vegan diet, but with less emphasis on raw foods and more emphasis on whole foods that are nonetheless prepared in a way to ensure minimum use of energy during preparation or preservation, for example through the practice of lacto fermentation and cooking at low temperatures under 70 °C (158 °F).

When lean & green food merges with air frying, it can make this diet much easier for people to follow. Air frying food cuts the cooking time in half and makes the food more nutritious.

The Lean and Green diet is a great diet to try. It can help you lose weight and eat healthy foods in the process. The diet practically makes the body burn fats much faster than carbohydrates.

Carbs will be there too, but at far lower levels than before. Foods rich in carbohydrates are the body's primary fuel or the brain's food. (Our bodies turn carbs into glucose.) Because there are hardly any carbohydrates in this diet, the body will have to find a substitute source of energy to keep itself alive.

Once the body realizes that it does not have enough carbohydrates to cover the calories it burns, it turns to fat reserves to provide the required energy. Before that time, the body was using only 15% of its fat reserves for energy—the ratio changes once you start this diet. You will burn fats at a relatively faster rate than fat reserves, and after that, it will burn fat at a relatively faster rate than fat reserves. In this way, the body will find a way to get the required amount of energy from its fat stores keeping the carbs and calories under control.

If you did not change your way of living altogether and added good fats to your diet, it could take carbohydrates. In that case, you might be waiting for at least a year before you will start losing weight with this diet. For you, it is still worth doing this diet. Even if it is yearlong, you will see a great improvement in your overall health. Therefore, when you ingest fats, instead of your body storing them as fat, they are more likely to be converted into a source of energy.

As fat reserves continue to be burned, the body will tend not to gain weight. This is excellent news because fat reserves are not very easy to get rid of completely.

If you ask a nutritionist about this diet, they will recommend it without a doubt. So, if you feel like cleansing your body and starting a diet that will keep you healthy, well-fed, and slender, this diet should be your primary choice.

Engaging into lean and green diet is a good idea to improve not only our health, but also our environment. One should eat less meat products and consume more of fresh fruits and vegetables in order to lower the risk for heart disease and cancer. The latter are mostly linked with meat consumption because of the nitrates located in processed meats. Fruits and vegetables are very low-calorie foods, but they are high in fiber content and rich in vitamins.

The vegetables and fruits that deserve to be consumed are the ones that are grown organically. It is very important to avoid processed foods since they contain a high percentage of fat. Green and lean diet is also linked with the environment preservation. By cutting down meat consumption by at least 50%, we save a lot from greenhouse gas emissions. Considering that meat production requires more energy, it causes more carbon dioxide emissions compared to vegetable production. Another advantage of green and lean diet is improved health care system and lower health problems cost.

Chapter 1. Lean and Green Foods

There are numerous categories of Lean and Green foods that you can eat while following this diet regime.

Green Foods
This section includes all kinds of vegetables that have been categorized from lower, moderate, and high in terms of carbohydrate content. One serving of vegetables should be at ½ cup unless otherwise specified.

Lower Carbohydrate - These are vegetables that contain low amounts of carbohydrates.

- A cup of green leafy vegetables, such as collard greens (raw), lettuce (green leaf, iceberg, butterhead, and romaine), spinach (raw), mustard greens, spring mix, bok choy (raw), and watercress.

- ½ cup of vegetables including cucumbers, celery, radishes, white mushroom, sprouts (mung bean, alfalfa), arugula, turnip greens, escarole, nopales, Swiss chard (raw), jalapeno, and bok choy (cooked).

Moderate Carbohydrate - These are vegetables that contain moderate amounts of carbohydrates.
Below are the types of vegetables that can be consumed in moderation:

- **½ cup of any of the following vegetables** such as asparagus, cauliflower, fennel bulb, eggplant, portabella mushrooms, kale, cooked spinach, summer squash (zucchini and scallop).

Higher Carbohydrates - Foods that are under this category contain a high amount of starch. Make sure to consume limited amounts of these vegetables.

- **½ cup of the following vegetables** like chayote squash, red cabbage, broccoli, cooked collard and mustard greens, green or wax beans, kohlrabi, kabocha squash, cooked leeks, any peppers, okra, raw scallion, summer squash such as straight neck and crookneck, tomatoes, spaghetti squash, turnips, jicama, cooked Swiss chard, and hearts of palm.

Lean Foods

Leanest Foods - These foods are considered to be the leanest as it has only up to 4 grams of total fat. Moreover, dieters should eat a 7-ounce cooked portion of these foods. Consume these foods with 1 healthy fat serving.

- **Fish:** Flounder, cod, haddock, grouper, Mahi, tilapia, tuna (yellowfin fresh or canned), and wild catfish.
- **Shellfish:** Scallops, lobster, crabs, shrimp
- **Game meat:** Elk, deer, buffalo
- **Ground turkey or other meat:** Should be 98% lean **Meatless alternatives:**14 egg whites, 2 cups egg
- substitute, 5 ounces seitan, 1 ½ cups 1% cottage cheese, and 12 ounces non-fat 0% Greek yogurt

Leaner Foods - These foods contain 5 to 9 grams of total fat. Consume these foods with 1 healthy fat serving. Make sure to consume only 6 ounces of a cooked portion of these foods daily:

- **Fish:** Halibut, trout, and swordfish
- **Chicken:** White meat such as breasts as long as the skin is removed
- **Turkey:** Ground turkey as long as it is 95% to 97% lean.
- **Meatless options:**2 whole eggs plus 4 egg whites, 2 whole eggs plus one cup egg substitute, 1 ½ cups 2% cottage cheese, and 12 ounces low fat 2% plain Greek yogurt

Lean Foods - These are foods that contain 10g to 20g total fat. When consuming these foods, there should be no serving of healthy fat. These include the following:

- **Fish:** Tuna (Bluefin steak), salmon, herring, farmed catfish, and mackerel
- **Lean beef:** Ground, steak, and roast
- **Lamb:** All cuts
- **Pork:** Pork chops, pork tenderloin, and all parts. Make sure to remove the skin
- **Ground turkey and other meats:**85% to 94% lean
- **Chicken:** Any dark meat

- **Meatless options:** 15 ounces extra-firm tofu, 3 whole eggs (up to two times per week), 4 ounces reduced-fat skim cheese, 8 ounces part-skim ricotta cheese, and 5 ounces tempeh

Healthy Fat Servings - Healthy fat servings are allowed under this diet. They should contain 5 grams of fat and less than grams of carbohydrates. Make sure that you add between 0 and 2 healthy fat servings daily. Below are the different healthy fat servings that you can eat:

- 1 teaspoon oil (any kind of oil)
- 1 tablespoon low carbohydrate salad dressing
- 2 tablespoons reduced-fat salad dressing
- 5 to 10 black or green olives
- 1 ½ ounce avocado
- 1/3-ounce plain nuts including peanuts, almonds, pistachios
- 1 tablespoon plain seeds such as chia, sesame, flax, and pumpkin seeds
- ½ tablespoon regular butter, mayonnaise, and margarine

Lean & Green Recipes

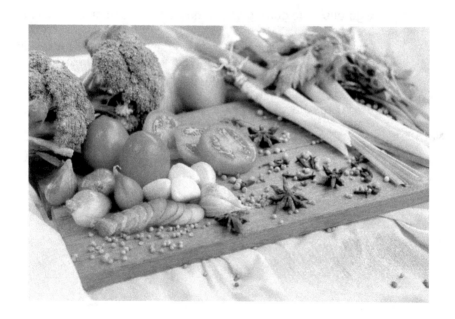

Chapter 2. Breakfast Recipes

1. Sun-Dried Tomato Garlic Bruschetta

Preparation Time: 10 Minutes
Cooking Time: 5 Minutes
Servings: 6
Ingredients:

- 2 Slices sourdough bread, toasted
- 1 Tsp. Chives, minced
- 1 Garlic clove, peeled
- 2 Tsp. Sun-dried tomatoes in olive oil, minced
- 1 Tsp. Olive oil

Directions:

1. Vigorously rub garlic clove on one side of each of the toasted bread slices
2. Spread equal portions of sun-dried tomatoes on the garlic side of the bread. Sprinkle chives and drizzle olive oil on top.
3. Pop both slices into an oven toaster, and cook until well heated through.
4. Place bruschetta on a plate. Serve warm.

Nutrition:

- Calories: 149 kcal
- Protein: 6.12g
- Fat: 2.99g
- Carbohydrates: 24.39g

2. Gingerbread Oatmeal Breakfast

Preparation Time: 10 Minutes
Cooking Time: 0 Minutes
Servings: 4
Ingredients:

- 1 cup steel-cut oats
- 4 cups drinking water
- Organic Maple syrup, to taste
- 1 Tsp. Ground cloves
- 1 ½ Tbsp. Ground cinnamon
- 1/8 Tsp. Nutmeg
- ¼ Tsp. Ground ginger
- ¼ Tsp. Ground coriander
- ¼ Tsp. Ground allspice
- ¼ Tsp. Ground cardamom
- Fresh mixed berries

Directions:

1. Cook the oats based on the package instructions. When it comes to a boil, reduce heat and simmer.
2. Stir in all the spices and continue cooking until cooked to desired doneness.
3. Serve in four serving bowls and drizzle with maple syrup and top with fresh berries.
4. Enjoy!

Nutrition:

- Calories: 87 kcal
- Protein: 5.82g
- Fat: 3.26g
- Carbohydrates: 18.22g

3. Oat Porridge With Cherry & Coconut

Preparation Time: 10 Minutes
Cooking Time: 0 Minutes
Servings: 3
Ingredients:

- 1 ½ Cups regular oats
- 3 cups coconut milk
- 4 Tbsp. Chia seed
- 3 Tbsp. Raw cacao
- Coconut shavings
- Dark chocolate shavings
- Fresh or frozen tart cherries
- A pinch of stevia, optional
- Maple syrup, to taste (optional)

Directions:

1. Combine the oats, milk, stevia, and cacao in a medium saucepan over medium heat and bring to a boil. Lower the heat, then simmer until the oats are cooked to desired doneness.
2. Divide the porridge among three serving bowls and top with dark chocolate, chia seeds, and coconut shavings, cherries, and a little drizzle of maple syrup.

Nutrition:

- Calories: 343 kcal
- Protein: 15.64g
- Fat: 12.78g
- Carbohydrates: 41.63g

4. Hash Browns

Preparation Time: 15 Minutes
Cooking Time: 15 Minutes
Servings: 4
Ingredients:

- 1 pound russet potatoes, peeled, processed using a grater
- Pinch of sea salt
- Pinch of black pepper, to taste
- 3 Tbsp. Olive oil

Directions:

1. Line a microwave safe-dish with paper towels. Spread shredded potatoes on top—microwave veggies on the highest heat setting for 2 minutes. Remove from heat.
2. Pour one tablespoon of oil into a non-stick skillet set over medium heat.
3. Cooking in batches, place a generous pinch of potatoes into the hot oil. Press down using the back of a spatula.
4. Cook for 3 minutes on every side, or until brown and crispy. Drain on paper towels—repeat the step for the remaining potatoes. Add more oil as needed.
5. Season with salt and pepper. Serve.

Nutrition:

- Calories: 200 kcal
- Protein: 4.03g
- Fat: 11.73g
- Carbohydrates: 20.49g

5. Apple Ginger and Rhubarb Muffins

Preparation Time: 15 Minutes
Cooking Time: 25 Minutes
Servings: 4
Ingredients:

- ½ Cup Finely ground almonds
- ¼ Cup Brown rice flour
- ½ Cup Buckwheat flour
- 1/8 Cup Unrefined raw sugar
- 2 Tbsp. Arrowroot flour
- 1 Tbsp. Linseed meal
- 2 Tbsp. Crystallized ginger, finely chopped
- ½ Tsp. Ground ginger
- ½ Tsp. Ground cinnamon
- 2 Tsp. Gluten-free baking powder
- A pinch of fine sea salt
- 1 small apple, peeled and finely diced
- 1 cup finely chopped rhubarb
- 1/3 cup almond/ rice milk
- 1 Large egg
- ¼ cup extra virgin olive oil
- 1 Tsp. Pure vanilla extract

Directions:

1. Set your oven to 350°F grease an eight-cup muffin tin and line with paper cases.
2. Combine the almond four, linseed meal, ginger, salt, and sugar in a mixing bowl. Sieve this mixture over the other flours, spices, and baking powder and use a whisk to combine well.
3. Stir in the apple and rhubarb in the flour mixture until evenly coated.
4. In a separate bowl, whisk the milk, vanilla, and egg, then pour it into the dry mixture. Stir until just combined — don't overwork the batter as this can yield very tough muffins.
5. Grease a muffin pan with oil. Scoop the mixture and top with a few slices of rhubarb. Bake for at least 25 minutes till they start turning golden or when an inserted toothpick emerges clean.
6. Take off from the oven and let sit for at least 5 minutes before transferring the muffins to a wire rack for further cooling.
7. Serve warm with a glass of squeezed juice.
8. Enjoy!

Nutrition:

- Calories: 325 kcal
- Protein: 6.32g
- Fat: 9.82g
- Carbohydrates: 55.71g

6. Anti-Inflammatory Breakfast Frittata

Preparation Time: 10 Minutes
Cooking Time: 40 Minutes
Servings: 4
Ingredients:

- 4 large eggs
- 6 Egg whites
- 450g Button mushrooms
- 450g Baby spinach
- 125g Firm tofu
- 1 Onion, chopped
- 1 Tbsp. Minced garlic
- ½ Tsp. Ground turmeric
- ½ Tsp. Cracked black pepper
- ¼ Cup water
- Kosher salt to taste

Directions:

1. Set your oven to 350°F.
2. Sauté the mushrooms in a little bit of extra virgin olive oil in a large non-stick ovenproof pan over medium heat. Add the onions once the mushrooms start turning golden and cook for 3 minutes until the onions become soft.
3. Stir in the garlic, then cook for at least 30 seconds until fragrant before adding the spinach. Pour in water, cover, and cook until the spinach becomes wilted for about 2 minutes.
4. Take off the lid and continue cooking up until the water evaporates. Now, combine the eggs, egg whites, tofu, pepper, turmeric, and salt in a bowl. When all the liquid has evaporated, pour in the egg mixture, let cook for about 2 minutes until the edges start setting, then transfer to the oven and bake for about 25 minutes or until cooked.
5. Take off from the oven, then let sit for at least 5 minutes before cutting it into quarters and serving.
6. Enjoy!

- **Tip:** Baby spinach and mushrooms boost the nutrient profile of the eggs to provide you with amazing anti-inflammatory benefits.

Nutrition:

- Calories: 521 kcal
- Protein: 29.13g
- Fat: 10.45g
- Carbohydrates: 94.94g

7. White and Green Quiche

Preparation Time: 10 Minutes
Cooking Time: 40 Minutes
Servings: 3
Ingredients:

- 3 Cups of fresh spinach, chopped
- 15 Large free-range eggs
- 3 Cloves of garlic, minced
- 5 White mushrooms, sliced
- 1 Small sized onion, finely chopped
- 1 ½ Teaspoon of baking powder
- Ground black pepper to taste
- 1 ½ Cups of coconut milk
- Ghee, as required to grease the dish
- Sea salt to taste

Directions:

1. Set the oven to 350°F.
2. Get a baking dish, then grease it with organic ghee.
3. Break all the eggs in a huge bowl, then whisk well.
4. Stir in coconut milk. Beat well
5. While you are whisking the eggs, start adding the remaining ingredients to them.
6. When all the ingredients are thoroughly blended, pour all of it into the prepared baking dish.
7. Bake for at least 40 minutes; up to the quiche is set in the middle.
8. Enjoy!

Nutrition:

- Calories: 608 kcal
- Protein: 20.28g
- Fat: 53.42g
- Carbohydrates: 16.88g

8. Yummy Steak Muffins

Preparation Time: 10 Minutes
Cooking Time: 20 Minutes
Servings: 4
Ingredients:

- 1 Cup red bell pepper, diced
- 2 Tablespoons of water
- 8 Ounces thin steak, cooked and finely chopped
- ¼ Teaspoon of sea salt
- Dash of freshly ground black pepper
- 8 Free-range eggs
- 1 Cup of finely diced onion

Directions:

1. Set the oven to 350°F
2. Take eight muffin tins and line them with parchment paper liners.
3. Get a large bowl and crack all the eggs in it.
4. Beat well the eggs.
5. Blend in all the remaining ingredients.
6. Spoon the batter into the arrange muffin tins. Fill three-fourth of each tin.
7. Put the muffin tins in the preheated oven for about 20 minutes, until the muffins are baked and set in the middle.
8. Enjoy!

Nutrition:

- Calories: 151 kcal
- Protein: 17.92g
- Fat: 7.32g
- Carbohydrates: 3.75g

9. Breakfast Sausage and Mushroom Casserole

Preparation Time: 20 Minutes
Cooking Time: 45 Minutes
Servings: 4
Ingredients:

- 450g of Italian sausage, cooked and crumbled
- ¾ Cup of coconut milk
- 8 Ounces of white mushrooms, sliced
- 1 Medium onion, finely diced
- 2 Tablespoons of organic ghee
- 6 Free-range eggs
- 600g of sweet potatoes
- 1 Red bell pepper, roasted
- 3/4 Tsp. of ground black pepper, divided
- 1 ½ Tsp. of sea salt, divided

Directions:

1. Peel and shred the sweet potatoes.
2. Take a bowl, fill it with ice-cold water, and soak the sweet potatoes in it. Set aside.
3. Peel the roasted bell pepper, remove its seeds and finely dice it.
4. Set the oven to 375°F.
5. Get a casserole baking dish and grease it with organic ghee.
6. Put a skillet over medium flame and cook the mushrooms in it. Cook until the mushrooms are crispy and brown.
7. Take the mushrooms out and mix them with the crumbled sausage.
8. Now sauté the onions in the same skillet. Cook up to the onions are soft and golden. This should take about 4–5 minutes.
9. Take the onions out and mix them in the sausage-mushroom mixture.
10. Add the diced bell pepper to the same mixture.

11. Mix well and set aside for a while.
12. Now drain the soaked shredded potatoes, put them on a paper towel, and pat dry.
13. Bring the sweet potatoes to a bowl and add about a teaspoon of salt and half a teaspoon of ground black pepper to it. Mix well and set aside.
14. Now take a large bowl and crack the eggs in it.
15. Break the eggs and then blend in the coconut milk.

16. Stir in the remaining black pepper and salt.
17. Take the greased casserole dish and spread the seasoned sweet potatoes evenly in the base of the dish.
18. Next, spread the sausage mixture evenly in the dish.
19. Finally, spread the egg mixture.
20. Now cover the casserole dish using a piece of aluminum foil.
21. Bake for 20-30 minutes. To check if the casserole is baked properly, insert a tester in the middle of the casserole, and it should come out clean.
22. Uncover the casserole dish and bake it again, uncovered for 5 -10 minutes, until the casserole is a little golden on the top.
23. Allow it to cool for 10 minutes.
24. Enjoy!

Nutrition:

- Calories: 598 kcal
- Protein: 28.65g
- Fat: 36.75g
- Carbohydrates: 48.01g

10. Mushroom Crêpes

Preparation Time: 1 Hour 30 minutes
Cooking Time: 30 Minutes
Servings: 6
Ingredients:

- 2 Eggs
- 3/4 Cup milk
- ½ Cup all-purpose flour
- 1/4 Teaspoon salt

For the filling:

- 3 Tablespoons all-purpose flour
- 2 cups of cremini mushrooms, sliced
- 3/4 cup chicken broth
- ½ Cup Parmesan cheese, grated
- 1/8 Teaspoon cayenne
- 1/8 Teaspoon nutmeg
- ¾ Cup milk
- 3 Garlic cloves, minced
- 2 Tablespoons of parsley (chopped)
- 6 Slices of deli-sliced cooked lean ham
- 1/4 Teaspoon of salt
- Freshly ground pepper

Directions:

1. Put and combine the salt and flour in a bowl. In another bowl, whisk the eggs and milk. Gradually combine the two mixtures until smooth. Leave for 15 minutes.
2. Spray a skillet using non-stick cooking spray and put it over medium heat. Stir the batter a little. Add 1/4 of the batter into the skillet. Tilt the skillet to form a thin and even crêpe. Cook for 1-2 minutes or until the bottom is golden and the top is set. Flip and cook for 20 seconds. Transfer to a plate.
3. Repeat the steps with the remaining batter. Loosely cover the cooked crêpes with plastic wrap.
4. Put all the ingredients together for filling in a saucepan on medium heat — flour, milk, cayenne, nutmeg, and pepper. Constantly whisk until thick or around 7 minutes. Remove from the stove. Stir in a tablespoon of parsley and cheese. Loosely cover to keep warm.
5. Spray a skillet using non-stick cooking spray and put over medium heat. Cook the garlic and mushrooms. Season with

salt. Cook for 6 minutes or until the mushrooms are soft. Add two tablespoons of sherry—Cook for a couple of minutes. Remove from the stove. Add the remaining parsley and stir.

6. Put the crêpes side by side on a flat surface. Spread a tablespoon of the sauce and two tablespoons of the cooked mushrooms. Roll up the crêpes and transfer them to a greased baking dish. Put all the sauce on top—Bake in the oven at 450°F for 15 minutes.

Nutrition:

- Calories: 232 kcal
- Protein: 16.51g
- Fat: 10.8g
- Carbohydrates: 16.25g

11. Beef Breakfast Casserole

Preparation Time: 10 Minutes
Cooking Time: 30 Minutes
Servings: 5
Ingredients:

- 1 Pound of ground beef, cooked
- 10 Eggs
- ½ Cup Pico de Gallo
- 1 Cup baby spinach
- ¼ Cup sliced black olives
- Freshly ground black pepper

Directions:

1. Preheat oven to 350 degrees Fahrenheit. Prepare a 9" glass pie plate with non-stick spray.
2. Whisk the eggs until frothy—season with salt and pepper.
3. Layer the cooked ground beef, Pico de Gallo, and spinach on the pie plate.
4. Slowly pour the eggs over the top.
5. Top with black olives.
6. Bake for at least 30 minutes until firm in the middle.
7. Slice into five pieces and serve.

Nutrition:

- Calories: 479 kcal
- Protein: 43.54g
- Fat: 30.59g
- Carbohydrates: 4.65g

12. Fantastic Spaghetti Squash With Cheese and Basil Pesto

Preparation Time: 10 Minutes
Cooking Time: 35 Minutes
Servings: 2
Ingredients:

- 1 Cup cooked spaghetti squash, drained
- Salt, to taste
- Freshly cracked black pepper, to taste
- ½ Tbsp. olive oil
- ¼ Cup ricotta cheese, unsweetened
- 2 oz. Fresh mozzarella cheese, cubed
- 1/8 Cup basil pesto

Directions:

1. Switch on the oven, then set its temperature to 375°F and let it preheat.
2. Meanwhile, take a medium bowl, add spaghetti squash in it and then season with salt and black pepper.
3. Take a casserole dish, grease it with oil, add squash mixture in it, top it with ricotta cheese and mozzarella cheese and bake for 10 minutes until cooked.
4. When done, remove the casserole dish from the oven, drizzle pesto on top and serve immediately.

Nutrition:

- Calories: 169
- Total Fat: 11.3g
- Total Carbs: 6.2g
- Protein: 11.9g
- Sugar: 0.1g
- Sodium 217mg

13. Ham and Veggie Frittata Muffins

Preparation Time: 10 Minutes
Cooking Time: 25 Minutes
Servings: 12
Ingredients:

- 5 Ounces thinly sliced ham
- 8 Large eggs
- 4 Tablespoons coconut oil
- ½ Yellow onion, finely diced
- 8 oz. Frozen spinach, thawed and drained
- 8 oz. Mushrooms, thinly sliced
- 1 Cup cherry tomatoes, halved
- ¼ Cup coconut milk (canned)
- 2 Tablespoons coconut flour
- Sea salt and pepper to taste

Directions:

1. Preheat oven to 375 degrees Fahrenheit.
2. In a medium skillet, warm the coconut oil on medium heat. Add the onion and cook until softened.
3. Add the mushrooms, spinach, and cherry tomatoes. Season with salt and pepper. Cook until the mushrooms have softened. About 5 minutes. Remove from heat and set aside.
4. In a huge bowl, beat the eggs together with coconut milk and coconut flour. Stir in the cooled veggie mixture.
5. Line each cavity of a 12 cavity muffin tin with the thinly sliced ham. Pour the egg mixture into each one and bake for 20 minutes.
6. Remove from oven and allow to cool for about 5 minutes before transferring to a wire rack.

   Tip: It's important to maximize the benefit of a vegetable-rich diet to eat a variety of colors, and these veggie-packed frittata
- muffins do just that. The onion, spinach, mushrooms, and cherry tomatoes provide a wide range of vitamins and nutrients and a healthy dose of fiber.

Nutrition:

- Calories: 125 kcal
- Protein: 5.96g
- Fat: 9.84g
- Carbohydrates: 4.48g

14. Cheesy Flax and Hemp Seeds Muffins

Preparation Time: 5 Minutes
Cooking Time: 30 Minutes
Servings: 2
Ingredients:

- 1/8 Cup flax seeds meal
- ¼ Cup raw hemp seeds
- ¼ Cup almond meal
- Salt, to taste
- ¼ Tsp. Baking powder
- 3 Organic eggs, beaten
- 1/8 Cup nutritional yeast flakes
- ¼ Cup cottage cheese, low-fat
- ¼ Cup grated parmesan cheese
- ¼ Cup scallion, sliced thinly
- 1 Tbsp. Olive oil

Directions:

1. Switch on the oven, then set it to 360°F and let it preheat.
2. Meanwhile, take two ramekins, grease them with oil, and set them aside until required.
3. Take a medium bowl, add flax seeds, hemp seeds, and almond meal, and then stir in salt and baking powder until mixed.
4. Crack eggs in another bowl, add yeast, cottage cheese, and parmesan, stir well until combined, and then stir this mixture into the almond meal mixture until incorporated.
5. Fold in scallions, then distribute the mixture between prepared ramekins and bake for 30 minutes until muffins are firm and the top is nicely golden brown.
6. When done, take out the muffins from the ramekins and let them cool completely on a wire rack.
7. For meal prepping, wrap each muffin with a paper towel and refrigerate for up to thirty-four days.
8. When ready to eat, reheat muffins in the microwave until hot and then serve.

Nutrition:

- Calories: 179
- Total Fat: 10.9g
- Total Carbs: 6.9g
- Protein: 15.4g
- Sugar: 2.3g
- Sodium: 311mg

15. Cheddar and Chive Souffles

Preparation Time: 10 Minutes
Cooking Time: 25 Minutes
Servings: 8
Ingredients:

- ½ Cup almond flour
- ¼ Cup chopped chives
- 1 Tsp. salt
- ½ Tsp. xanthan gum
- 1 Tsp. ground mustard
- ¼ Tsp. cayenne pepper
- ½ Tsp. cracked black pepper
- ¾ Cup heavy cream
- 2 Cups shredded cheddar cheese
- ½ Cup baking powder
- 6 Organic eggs, separated

Directions:

1. Switch on the oven, then set its temperature to 350°F and let it preheat.
2. Take a medium bowl, add flour in it, add remaining ingredients, except for baking powder and eggs, and whisk until combined.
3. Separate egg yolks and egg whites between two bowls, add egg yolks in the flour mixture, and whisk until incorporated.
4. Add baking powder into the egg whites and beat with an electric mixer until stiff peaks form, and then stir egg whites into the flour mixture until well mixed.
5. Divide the batter evenly between eight ramekins and then bake for 25 minutes until done.
6. Serve straight away or store in the refrigerator until ready to eat.

Nutrition:

- Calories: 288
- Total Fat: 21g
- Total Carbs: 3g
- Protein: 14g

16. Shirataki Pasta With Avocado and Cream

Preparation Time: 10 Minutes
Cooking Time: 6 Minutes
Servings: 2
Ingredients:

- ½ Packet of shirataki noodles, cooked
- ½ Avocado
- ½ Tsp. cracked black pepper
- ½ Tsp. salt
- ½ Tsp. dried basil
- 1/8 Cup heavy cream

Directions:

1. Place a medium pot half full with water over medium heat, bring it to boil, then add noodles and cook for 2 minutes.
2. Then drain the noodles and set them aside until required.
3. Place avocado in a bowl, mash it with a fork,
4. Mash avocado in a bowl, transfer it to a blender, add remaining ingredients, and pulse until smooth.
5. Take a frying pan, place it over medium heat and when hot, add noodles in it, pour in the avocado mixture, stir well and cook for 2 minutes until hot.
6. Serve straight away.

Nutrition:

- Calories: 131
- Total Fat: 12.6g
- Total Carbs: 4.9g
- Protein: 1.2g
- Sugar: 0.3g
- Sodium: 588mg

17. Mango Granola

Preparation Time: 10 Minutes
Cooking Time: 30 Minutes
Servings: 4
Ingredients:

- 2 Cups rolled oats
- 1 Cup dried mango, chopped
- ½ Cup almonds, roughly chopped
- ½ Cup nuts
- ½ Cup dates, roughly chopped
- 3 Tbsp. Sesame seeds
- 2 Tsp. Cinnamon
- 2/3 Cups agave nectar
- 2 Tbsp. Coconut oil
- 2 Tbsp. Water

Directions:

1. Set the oven at 320°F
2. In a large bowl, put the oats, almonds, nuts, sesame seeds, dates, and cinnamon, then mix well.
3. Meanwhile, heat a saucepan over medium heat, pour in the agave syrup, coconut oil, and water.
4. Stir and let it cook for at least 3 minutes or until the coconut oil has melted.
5. Gradually pour the syrup mixture into the bowl with the oats and nuts and stir well, ensure that all the ingredients are coated with the syrup.
6. Transfer the granola to a baking sheet lined with parchment paper and place in the oven to bake for 20 minutes.
7. After 20 minutes, take off the tray from the oven and lay the chopped dried mango on top. Put back in the oven, then bake again for another 5 minutes.
8. Let the granola cool to room temperature before serving or placing it in an airtight container for storage. The shelf life of the granola will last up to 2-3 weeks.

Nutrition:

- Calories: 434 kcal
- Protein: 13.16g
- Fat: 28.3g
- Carbohydrates: 55.19g

18. Blueberry & Cashew Waffles

Preparation Time: 15 Minutes
Cooking Time: 4-5 Minutes
Servings: 5
Ingredients:

- 1 Cup raw cashews
- 3 Tablespoons coconut flour
- 1 Tsp. Baking soda
- Salt, to taste
- ½ Cup unsweetened almond milk
- 3 Organic eggs
- ¼ Cup coconut oil, melted
- 3 Tablespoons organic honey
- ½ Teaspoon organic vanilla flavor
- 1 Cup fresh blueberries

Directions:

1. Preheat the waffle iron, after which grease it.
2. In a mixer, add cashews and pulse till flour-like consistency forms.
3. Transfer the cashew flour to a big bowl.
4. Add almond flour, baking soda, and salt and mix well.
5. In another bowl, put the remaining ingredients and beat till well combined.
6. Put the egg mixture into the flour mixture, then mix till well combined.
7. Fold in blueberries.
8. In the preheated waffle iron, add the required amount of mixture.
9. Cook for around 4-5 minutes.
10. Repeat with the remaining mixture.

Nutrition:

- Calories: 432
- Fat: 32
- Carbohydrates: 32g
- Protein: 13g

19. Tomato and Avocado Omelet

Preparation Time: 5 Minutes
Cooking Time: 5 Minutes
Servings: 1
Ingredients:

- 2 Eggs
- ¼ avocado, diced
- 4 Cherry tomatoes, halved
- 1 tablespoon cilantro, chopped
- Squeezed lime juice
- Pinch of salt

Directions:

1. Put together the avocado, tomatoes, cilantro, lime juice, and salt in a small bowl, then mix well and set aside.
2. Warm a medium non-stick skillet on medium heat, whisk the eggs until frothy and add to the pan. Move the eggs around gently with a rubber spatula until they begin to set.
3. Scatter the avocado mixture over half of the omelet. Remove from heat, and slide the omelet onto a plate as you fold it in half.
4. Serve immediately.

Nutrition:

- Calories: 433 kcal
- Protein: 25.55g
- Fat: 32.75g
- Carbohydrates: 10.06g

20. Vegan-Friendly Banana Bread

Preparation Time: 15 Minutes
Cooking Time: 40 Minutes
Servings: 4-6
Ingredients:

- 2 Ripe bananas, mashed
- 1/3 Cup brewed coffee
- 3 Tbsp. Chia seeds
- 6 Tbsp. Water
- ½ Cup soft vegan butter
- ½ Cup maple syrup
- 2 Cups flour
- 2 Tsp. Baking powder
- 1 Tsp. Cinnamon powder
- 1 Tsp. Allspice
- ½ Tsp. Salt

Directions:

1. Set the oven at 350°F.
2. Bring the chia seeds in a small bowl, then soak them with 6 Tbsp. of water. Stir well and set aside.
3. In a mixing bowl, mix using a hand mixer the vegan butter and maple syrup until it turns fluffy. Add the chia seeds along with the mashed bananas.
4. Mix well, and then add the coffee.
5. Meanwhile, sift all the dry ingredients (flour, baking powder, cinnamon powder, allspice, and salt) and then gradually add into the bowl with the wet ingredients.
6. Combine the ingredients well, and then pour over a baking pan lined with parchment paper.
7. Place in the oven to bake for at least 30-40 minutes or until the toothpick comes out clean after inserting in the bread.
8. Allow the bread to cool before serving.

Nutrition:

- Calories: 371 kcal
- Protein: 5.59g
- Fat: 16.81g
- Carbohydrates: 49.98g

Chapter 3. Side Dish Recipes

21. Plant-Powered Pancakes

Preparation Time: 5 Minutes
Cooking Time: 15 Minutes
Servings: 8
Ingredients:

- 1 Cup whole-wheat flour
- 1 Teaspoon baking powder
- ½ Teaspoon ground cinnamon
- 1 Cup plant-based milk
- ½ Cup unsweetened applesauce
- 1/4 Cup maple syrup
- 1 Teaspoon vanilla extract

Directions:

1. In a large bowl, combine the flour, baking powder, and cinnamon.
2. Stir in the milk, applesauce, maple syrup, and vanilla until no dry flour is left and the batter is smooth.
3. Heat a large, nonstick skillet or griddle over medium heat. For each pancake, pour 1/4 cup of batter onto the hot skillet. Once bubbles form over the top of the pancake and the sides begin to brown, flip and cook for 1 or 2 minutes more.
4. Repeat until the entire batter is used, and serve.

Nutrition:

- Fat: 2g
- Carbohydrates: 44g
- Fiber: 5g
- Protein: 5g

22. Hemp Seed Porridge

Preparation Time: 5 Minutes
Cooking Time: 5 Minutes
Servings: 6
Ingredients:

- 3 Cups cooked hemp seed
- 1 Packet Stevia
- 1 Cup coconut milk

Directions:

1. In a saucepan, mix the seeds and the coconut milk over moderate heat for about 5 minutes as you stir it constantly.
2. Remove the pan from the burner, then add the Stevia. Stir.
3. Serve in 6 bowls.
4. Enjoy.

Nutrition:

- Calories: 236 kcal
- Fat: 1.8g
- Carbs: 48.3g
- Protein: 7g

23. Walnut Crunch Banana Bread

Preparation Time: 5 minutes
Cooking Time: 1 hour and 30 minutes
Servings: 1
Ingredients:

- 4 Ripe bananas
- 1/4 Cup maple syrup
- 1 Tablespoon apple cider vinegar
- 1 Teaspoon vanilla extract
- 1½ Cups whole-wheat flour
- ½ Teaspoon ground cinnamon
- ½ Teaspoon baking soda
- 1/4 Cup walnut pieces (optional)

Directions:

1. Preheat the oven to 350°F.
2. In a large bowl, use a fork or mixing spoon to mash the bananas until they reach a puréed consistency (small bits of banana are acceptable). Stir in the maple syrup, apple cider vinegar, and vanilla.
3. Stir in the flour, cinnamon, and baking soda. Fold in the walnut pieces (if using).
4. Gently pour the batter into a loaf pan, filling it no more than three-quarters of the way full, bake for 1 hour, or until you can stick a knife into the middle and it comes out clean.
5. Remove from the oven and allow cooling on the countertop for a minimum of 30 minutes before serving.

Nutrition:

- Fat: 1g
- Carbohydrates: 40g
- Fiber: 5g
- Protein: 4g

24. Mini Mac in a Bowl

Preparation Time: 5 Minutes
Cooking Time: 15 Minutes
Servings: 1
Ingredients:

- 5 Ounces of lean ground beef
- 2 Tablespoons of diced white or yellow onion.
- 1/8 Teaspoon of onion powder
- 1/8 Teaspoon of white vinegar
- 1 Ounce of dill pickle slices
- 1 Teaspoon sesame seed
- 3 Cups of shredded romaine lettuce
- Cooking spray
- 2 Tablespoons reduced-fat shredded cheddar cheese
- 2 Tablespoons of wish-bone light thousand island as dressing

Directions:

1. Place a lightly greased small skillet on fire to heat.
2. Add your onion to cook for about 2-3 minutes.
3. Next, add the beef and allow cooking until it's brown.
4. Next, mix your vinegar and onion powder with the dressing.
5. Finally, top the lettuce with the cooked meat and sprinkle cheese on it; add your pickle slices.
6. Drizzle the mixture with the sauce and sprinkle the sesame seeds.
7. Your mini mac in a bowl is ready to eat.

Nutrition:

- Calories: 150
- Protein: 21g
- Carbohydrates: 32g
- Fats: 19g

25. Mini Zucchini Bites

Preparation Time: 10 Minutes
Cooking Time: 10 Minutes
Servings: 6
Ingredients:

- 1 Zucchini, cut into thick circles
- 3 Cherry tomatoes, halved
- ½ Cup parmesan cheese, grated
- Salt and pepper to taste
- 1 Tsp. Chives, chopped

Directions:

1. Preheat the oven to 390 degrees F.
2. Add wax paper to a baking sheet.
3. Arrange the zucchini pieces.
4. Add the cherry halves to each zucchini slice.
5. Add parmesan cheese, chives, and sprinkle with salt and pepper.
6. Bake for 10 minutes. Serve.

Nutrition:

- Fat: 1.0g
- Cholesterol: 5.0mg
- Sodium: 400.3mg
- Potassium: 50.5mg
- Carbohydrates: 7.3g

26. Lean and Green Smoothie 2

Preparation Time: 5 Minutes
Cooking Time: 0 Minutes
Servings: 1
Ingredients:

- Six kale leaves
- Two peeled oranges
- 2 Cups of mango kombucha
- 2 Cups of chopped pineapple
- 2 Cups of water

Directions:

1. Break up the oranges, place them in the blender.
2. Add the mango kombucha, chopped pineapple, and kale leaves into the blender.
3. Blend everything until it is smooth.
4. Smoothie is ready to be taken.

Nutrition:

- Calories: 81
- Protein: 2g
- Carbohydrates: 19g
- Fats: 1g

27. Mushroom & Spinach Omelet

Preparation Time: 20 Minutes
Cooking Time: 20 Minutes
Servings: 3
Ingredients:

- 2 Tablespoons butter, divided
- 6-8 Fresh mushrooms, sliced, 5 ounces
- Chives, chopped, optional
- Salt and pepper, to taste
- 1 Handful baby spinach, about ½ ounce
- Pinch garlic powder
- 4 Eggs, beaten
- 1-ounce Shredded swiss cheese

Directions:

1. In a very large saucepan, sauté the mushrooms in one tablespoon of butter until soft—season with salt, pepper, and garlic.
2. Remove the mushrooms from the pan and keep warm. Heat the remaining tablespoon of butter in the same skillet over medium heat.
3. Beat the eggs with a little salt and pepper and add to the hot butter. Turn the pan over to coat the entire bottom of the pan with the beaten eggs. Once the egg is almost done, place the cheese over the middle of the tortilla.
4. Fill the cheese with spinach leaves and hot mushrooms. Let cook for about a minute for the spinach to start to wilt. Fold the empty side of the tortilla carefully over the filling and slide it onto a plate and sprinkle with chives, if desired.
5. Alternatively, you can make two tortillas using half the mushroom, spinach, and cheese filling in each.

Nutrition:

- Calories: 321
- Fat: 26g
- Protein: 19g
- Carbohydrate: 4g
- Dietary Fiber: 1g

28. Whole-Wheat Blueberry Muffins

Preparation Time: 5 Minutes
Cooking Time: 25 Minutes
Servings: 8
Ingredients:

- ½ Cup plant-based milk
- ½ Cup unsweetened applesauce
- ½ Cup maple syrup
- 1 Teaspoon vanilla extract
- 2 Cups whole-wheat flour
- ½ Teaspoon baking soda
- 1 Cup blueberries

Directions:

1. Preheat the oven to 375°F.
2. In a large bowl, mix the milk, applesauce, maple syrup, and vanilla.
3. Stir in the flour and baking soda until no dry flour is left and the batter is smooth.
4. Gently fold in the blueberries until they are evenly distributed throughout the batter.
5. In a muffin tin, fill eight muffin cups with three-quarters full of batter.
6. Bake for 25 minutes, or until you can stick a knife into the center of a muffin and it comes out clean. Allow cooling before serving.

Tip: Both frozen and fresh blueberries will work great in this recipe. The only difference will be that muffins using fresh blueberries will cook slightly quicker than those using frozen.
Nutrition:

- Fat: 1g
- Carbohydrates: 45g
- Fiber: 2g
- Protein: 4g

29. Sweet Cashew Cheese Spread

Preparation Time: 5 Minutes
Cooking Time: 5 Minutes
Servings: 10 Servings
Ingredients:

- Stevia (5 drops)
- Cashews (2 cups, raw)
- Water (½ cup)

Directions:

1. Soak the cashews overnight in water.
2. Next, drain the excess water then transfer cashews to a food processor.
3. Add in the stevia and the water.
4. Process until smooth.
5. Serve chilled. Enjoy.

Nutrition:

- Fat: 7g
- Cholesterol: 0mg
- Sodium: 12.6mg
- Carbohydrates: 5.7g

30. Mouthwatering Tuna Melts

Preparation Time: 15 Minutes
Cooking Time: 20 Minutes
Servings: 8
Ingredients:

- 1/8 Teaspoon Salt
- 1/3 Cup onion, chopped
- 16 1/3 Ounces Biscuits, refrigerated, flaky layers
- 10 Ounces Tuna, water-packed, drained
- 1/3 Cup Mayonnaise
- 1/8 Teaspoon Pepper
- 4 Ounces Cheddar cheese, shredded
- Tomato, chopped
- Sour cream
- Lettuce, shredded

Directions:

1. Preheat the air fryer at 325 degrees Fahrenheit.
2. Put some cooking spray onto a cookie sheet.
3. Mix tuna with mayonnaise, pepper, salt, and onion.
4. Separate the dough, so you have eight biscuits; press each into 5-inch rounds.
5. Arrange four biscuit rounds on the sheet. Fill at the center with tuna mixture before topping with cheese. Cover with the remaining biscuit rounds and press to seal.
6. Air-fry for fifteen to twenty minutes, slice each sandwich into halves. Serve each piece topped with lettuce, tomato, and sour cream.

Nutrition:

- Calories: 320
- Fat: 10g
- Protein: 10g
- Carbohydrates: 20g

31. Easiest Tuna Cobbler Ever

Preparation Time: 15 Minutes
Cooking Time: 25 Minutes
Servings: 4
Ingredients:

- Water, cold (1/3 cup)
- Tuna, canned, drained (10 ounces)
- Sweet pickle relish (2 tablespoons)
- Mixed vegetables, frozen (1 ½ cups)
- Soup, cream of chicken, condensed (10 ¾ ounces)
- Pimientos, sliced, drained (2 ounces)
- Lemon juice (1 teaspoon)
- Paprika

Directions:

1. Preheat the air fryer at 375 degrees Fahrenheit.
2. Mist cooking spray into a round casserole (1 ½ quart).
3. Mix the frozen vegetables with milk, soup, lemon juice, relish, pimientos, and tuna in a saucepan— cook for 8 minutes over medium heat.
4. Fill the casserole with the tuna mixture.
5. Combine the biscuit mix with cold water to form a soft dough. Beat for half a minute before pouring four spoonfuls into the casserole.
6. Dust the dish with paprika before air-frying for twenty to twenty-five minutes.

Nutrition:

- Calories: 320
- Fat: 10g
- Protein: 20g
- Carbohydrates: 30g

32. Lean and Green Smoothie 1

Preparation Time: 5 Minutes
Cooking Time: 0 Minutes
Servings: 1
Ingredients:

- 2 ½ Cups of kale leaves
- 3/4 Cup of chilled apple juice
- 1 Cup of cubed pineapple
- ½ Cup of frozen green grapes
- ½ Cup of chopped apple

Directions:

1. Place the pineapple, apple juice, apple, frozen green grapes, and kale leaves in a blender.
2. Cover and blend until it's smooth.
3. Smoothie is ready and can be garnished with halved grapes if you wish.

Nutrition:

- Calories: 81
- Protein: 2g
- Carbohydrates: 19g
- Fats: 1g

33. Deliciously Homemade Pork Buns

Preparation Time: 20 Minutes
Cooking Time: 25 Minutes
Servings: 8
Ingredients:

- 3 Pieces green onions, sliced thinly
- 1 Egg, beaten
- 1 Cup of pulled pork, diced, w/ barbecue sauce
- 16 1/3 Ounces buttermilk biscuits, refrigerated
- 1 Teaspoon soy sauce

Directions:

1. Preheat the air fryer at 325 degrees Fahrenheit.
2. Use parchment paper to line your baking sheet.
3. Combine pork with green onions.
4. Separate and press the dough to form 8 four-inch rounds.
5. Fill each biscuit round's center with two tablespoons of pork mixture. Cover with the dough edges and seal by pinching. Arrange the buns on the sheet and brush with a mixture of soy sauce and egg.
6. Cook in the air fryer for twenty to twenty-five minutes.

Nutrition:

- Calories: 240
- Fat: 0g
- Protein: 0g
- Carbohydrates: 20g

34. Yogurt Garlic Chicken

Preparation Time: 30 Minutes
Cooking Time: 60 Minutes
Servings: 6
Ingredients:

- 6 Pieces pita bread rounds, halved
- 1 Cup English cucumber, sliced thinly, w/ each slice halved

Chicken & vegetables:

- 3 Tablespoons olive oil
- ½ Teaspoon of black pepper, freshly ground
- 20 Ounces chicken thighs, skinless, boneless
- 1 Piece bell pepper, red, sliced into half-inch portions
- 4 Pieces garlic cloves, chopped finely
- ½ Teaspoon cumin, ground
- 1 Piece red onion, medium, sliced into half-inch wedges
- ½ Cup yogurt, plain, fat-free
- 2 Tablespoons lemon juice
- 1 ½ Teaspoons salt
- ½ Teaspoon red pepper flakes, crushed
- ½ Teaspoon allspice, ground
- 1 Piece bell pepper, yellow, sliced into half-inch portions

Yogurt sauce:

- 2 Tablespoons olive oil
- 1/4 Teaspoon salt
- 1 Tablespoon parsley, flat-leaf, chopped finely
- 1 Cup yogurt, plain, fat-free
- 1 Tablespoon lemon juice, fresh
- 1 Piece garlic clove, chopped finely

Directions:

1. Mix the yogurt (½ cup), garlic cloves (4 pieces), olive oil (1 tablespoon), salt (1 teaspoon), lemon juice (2 tablespoons), pepper (1/4 teaspoon), allspice, cumin, and pepper flakes. Stir in the chicken and coat well. Cover and marinate in the fridge for two hours.
2. Preheat the air fryer at 400 degrees Fahrenheit.
3. Grease a rimmed baking sheet (18x13-inch) with cooking spray.

4. Toss the bell peppers and onion with remaining olive oil (2 tablespoons), pepper (1/4 teaspoon), and salt (½ teaspoon).
5. Arrange veggies on the baking sheets left side and the marinated chicken thighs (drain first) on the right side—cook in the air fryer for twenty-five to thirty minutes.
6. Mix the yogurt sauce ingredients.
7. Slice air-fried chicken into half-inch strips.
8. Top each pita round with chicken strips, roasted veggies, cucumbers, and yogurt sauce.

Nutrition:

- Calories: 380
- Fat: 10g
- Protein: 20g
- Carbohydrates: 30g

35. Tuna Spinach Casserole

Preparation Time: 30 Minutes
Cooking Time: 25 Minutes
Servings: 8
Ingredients:

- 18 Ounces mushroom soup, creamy
- ½ Cup milk
- 12 Ounces white tuna, solid, in water, drained
- 8 Ounces crescent dinner rolls, refrigerated
- 8 Ounces egg noodles, wide, uncooked
- 8 Ounces cheddar cheese, shredded
- 9 Ounces spinach, chopped, frozen, thawed, drained
- 2 Teaspoons lemon peel grated

Directions:

1. Preheat the oven to 350 degrees Fahrenheit.
2. Put cooking spray onto a glass baking dish (11x7-inch).
3. Follow package directions in cooking and draining the noodles.
4. Stir the cheese (1 ½ cups) and soup together in a skillet heated on medium. Once cheese melts, stir in your noodles, milk, spinach, tuna, and lemon peel. Once bubbling, pour into the prepped dish.
5. Unroll the dough and sprinkle with remaining cheese (½ cup). Roll up dough and pinch at the edges to seal. Slice into eight portions and place over the tuna mixture.
6. Put all in the Air-fry mode for twenty to twenty-five minutes.

Nutrition:

- Calories: 400
- Fat: 10g
- Protein: 20g
- Carbohydrates: 30g

36. Lean and Green Chicken Pesto Pasta

Preparation Time: 5 Minutes
Cooking Time: 15 Minutes
Servings: 1
Ingredients:

- 3 Cups of raw kale leaves
- 2 Tbsp. of olive oil
- 2 Cups of fresh basil
- 1/4 teaspoon salt
- 3 Tbsp. Lemon juice
- Three garlic cloves
- 2 Cups of cooked chicken breast
- 1 Cup of baby spinach
- 6 Ounces of uncooked chicken pasta
- 3 Ounces of diced fresh mozzarella
- Basil leaves or red pepper flakes to garnish

Directions:

1. Start by making the pesto; add the kale, lemon juice, basil, garlic cloves, olive oil, and salt to a blender and blend until smooth.
2. Add salt and pepper to taste.
3. Cook the pasta and strain off the water. Reserve 1/4 cup of the liquid.
4. Get a bowl and mix everything, the cooked pasta, pesto, diced chicken, spinach, mozzarella, and the reserved pasta liquid.
5. Sprinkle the mixture with additional chopped basil or red paper flakes (optional).
6. Now your salad is ready. You may serve it warm or chilled. Also, it can be taken as a salad mix-ins or as a side dish. Leftovers should be stored in the refrigerator inside an air-tight container for 3-5 days.

Nutrition:

- Calories: 244
- Protein: 20.5g
- Carbohydrates: 22.5g
- Fats: 10g

37. Open-Face Egg Sandwiches With Cilantro-Jalapeño Spread

Preparation Time: 20 Minutes
Cooking Time: 10 Minutes
Servings: 2
Ingredients:
For the cilantro and jalapeño spread:

- 1 Cup filled up fresh cilantro leaves and stems (about a bunch)
- 1 Jalapeño pepper, seeded and roughly chopped
- ½ Cup extra-virgin olive oil
- ¼ Cup pepitas (hulled pumpkin seeds), raw or roasted
- 2 Garlic cloves, thinly sliced
- 1 Tablespoon freshly squeezed lime juice
- 1 Teaspoon kosher salt

For the eggs:

- 4 Large eggs
- ¼ Cup milk
- ¼ to ½ Teaspoon Kosher Salt
- 2 Tablespoons butter

For the sandwich:

- 2 Bread slices
- 1 Tablespoon butter
- 1 Avocado, halved, pitted, and divided into slices
- Microgreens or sprouts for garnish

Directions:
To make the cilantro and jalapeño spread:

1. In a food processor, combine the cilantro, jalapeño, oil, pepitas, garlic, lime juice, and salt. Whirl until smooth. Refrigerate it if preparing in advance; otherwise, set it aside.

To make the eggs:

1. In a medium bowl, whisk the eggs, milk, and salt.
2. Dissolve the butter in a skillet over low heat, swirling to coat the bottom of the pan. Pour in the whisked eggs.
3. Cook until they begin to set, using a heatproof spatula, push them to the sides, allowing the uncooked portions to run into the bottom of the skillet.

4. Continue until the eggs are set.

To assemble the sandwiches:

1. Toast the bread and spread it with butter.
2. Spread a spoonful of the cilantro-jalapeño spread on each piece of toast. Top each with scrambled eggs.
3. Arrange avocado over each sandwich and garnish with microgreens.

Nutrition:

- Calories: 711
- Total fat: 4g
- Cholesterol: 54mg
- Fiber: 12g
- Protein: 12g
- Sodium: 327mg

38. Lemony Parmesan Salmon

Preparation Time: 10 Minutes
Cooking Time: 25 Minutes
Servings: 4
Ingredients:

- 2 Tablespoons butter, melted
- 2 Tablespoons green onions, sliced thinly
- 3/4 Cups breadcrumbs, white, fresh
- 1/4 Teaspoon thyme leaves, dried
- 1 Piece salmon fillet, 1 ¼-pound
- 1/4 Teaspoon salt
- 1/4 Cup parmesan cheese, grated
- 2 Teaspoons lemon peel, grated

Directions:

1. Preheat the oven to 350 degrees Fahrenheit.
2. Mist cooking spray onto a baking pan (shallow). Fill with pat-dried salmon—brush salmon with butter (1 tablespoon) before sprinkling with salt.
3. Combine the breadcrumbs with onions, thyme, lemon peel, cheese, and remaining butter (1 tablespoon).
4. Cover salmon with the breadcrumb mixture. Air-fry for fifteen to twenty-five minutes.

Nutrition:

- Calories: 290
- Fat: 10g
- Protein: 30g
- Carbohydrates: 0g

39. Chicken Omelet

Preparation Time: 5 Minutes
Cooking Time: 15 Minutes
Servings: 1
Ingredients:

- 2 Bacon slices; cooked and crumbled
- 2 Eggs
- 1 Tablespoon homemade mayonnaise
- 1 Tomato; chopped.
- 1-Ounce rotisserie chicken; shredded
- 1 Teaspoon mustard
- 1 Small avocado; pitted, peeled, and chopped.
- Salt and black pepper, to the taste.

Directions:

1. In a bowl, mix eggs with some salt and pepper and whisk gently.
2. Heat up a pan over medium heat; spray with some cooking oil, add eggs and cook your omelet for 5 minutes
3. Add chicken, avocado, tomato, bacon, mayo, and mustard on one half of the omelet.
4. Fold omelet, cover the pan and cook for 5 minutes more
5. Transfer to a plate and serve

Nutrition:

- Calories: 400
- Fat: 32
- Fiber: 6
- Carbs: 4
- Protein: 25

40. Pepper Pesto Lamb

Preparation Time: 15 Minutes
Cooking Time: 1 Hour 15 Minutes
Servings: 12
Ingredients:
For the Pesto:

- 1/4 Cup rosemary leaves, fresh
- 3 Pieces garlic cloves
- 3/4 Cups parsley, fresh, packed firmly
- 1/4 Cup mint leaves, fresh
- 2 Tablespoons olive oil

Lamb:

- 7 ½ Ounces red bell peppers, roasted, drained
- 5 Pounds leg of lamb, boneless, rolled
- 2 Teaspoons seasoning, lemon pepper

Directions:

1. Preheat the oven to 325 degrees Fahrenheit.
2. Mix the pesto ingredients in the food processor.
3. Unroll the lamb and cover the cut side with pesto. Top with roasted peppers before rolling up the lamb and tying with kitchen twine.
4. Coat lamb with seasoning (lemon pepper) and air-fry for one hour.

Nutrition:

- Calories: 310
- Fat: 10g
- Protein: 40.0g
- Carbohydrates: 0g

41. Best Whole Wheat Pancakes

Preparation Time: 10 Minutes
Cooking Time: 20 Minutes
Servings: 1
Ingredients:

- 3/4 Tablespoons ground flaxseed
- 2 Tablespoons warm water
- ½ Cups whole wheat pastry flour
- 1/8 Cup rye flour
- ½ Tablespoons double-acting baking powder
- 1/4 Teaspoon ground cinnamon
- 1/8 Teaspoon ground ginger
- 1 Cup unsweetened nondairy milk
- 3/4 Tablespoons pure maple syrup
- 1/4 Teaspoon vanilla extract

Directions:

1. Mix the warm water and flaxseed in a large bowl. Set aside for at least 5 minutes.
2. Whisk together the pastry and rye flours, baking powder, cinnamon, and ginger.
3. Whisk together the milk, maple syrup, and vanilla in a large bowl. Make use of a spatula, fold the wet ingredients into the dry ingredients. Fold in the soaked flaxseed until fully incorporated.
4. Heat a large skillet or nonstick griddle over medium-high heat.
5. Working in batches, three to four pancakes at a time, add 1/4-cup portions of batter to the hot skillet.
6. Cook for 3 to 4 minutes on each side until golden brown or no liquid batter is visible.

Nutrition:

- Calories: 301
- Fat: 4g
- Protein: 10g
- Carbohydrates: 57g
- Fiber: 10g

42. Spiced Pumpkin Muffins

Preparation Time: 15 Minutes
Cooking Time: 20 Minutes
Servings: 1
Ingredients:

- 1/6 Tablespoons ground flaxseed
- ¼4 Cup of water
- 1/8 Cups whole wheat flour
- 1/6 Teaspoons baking powder
- 5/6 Teaspoons ground cinnamon
- 1/12 Teaspoon baking soda
- 1/12 Teaspoon ground ginger
- 1/16 Teaspoon ground nutmeg
- 1/32 Teaspoon ground cloves
- 1/6 Cup pumpkin puree
- 1/12 Cup pure maple syrup
- ¼4 Cup unsweetened applesauce
- ¼4 Cup unsweetened nondairy milk
- ½ Teaspoons vanilla extract

Directions:

1. Preheat the oven to 350°F. Line a 12-cup metal muffin pan with parchment paper liners, or use a silicone muffin pan.
2. First, mix the flaxseed and water in a large bowl, then keep it aside.
3. In a medium bowl, stir together the flour, baking powder, cinnamon, baking soda, ginger, nutmeg, and cloves.
4. In a medium bowl, stir up the maple syrup, pumpkin puree, applesauce, milk, and vanilla. Pour the wet ingredients into the dry ingredients making use of a spatula.
5. Fold the soaked flaxseed into the batter until evenly combined, but do not over mix the batter, or your muffins will become dense. Spoon about 1/4 cup of batter per muffin into your prepared muffin pan.
6. Bake for 18 to 20 minutes, or until a toothpick inserted into the center of a muffin comes out clean. Remove the muffins from the pan.
7. Transfer to a wire rack for cooling.
8. Store in an airtight container that is at room temperature.

Nutrition:

- Calories: 115
- Fat: 1g
- Protein: 3g
- Carbohydrates: 25g
- Fiber: 3g

Chapter 4. Salads

43. Blueberry Cantaloupe Avocado Salad

Preparation Time: 5 Minutes
Cooking Time: 0 Minutes
Servings: 2
Ingredients:

- 1 Diced cantaloupe
- 2–3 Chopped avocados
- 1 Package of blueberries
- ¼ Cup olive oil
- 1/8 Cup balsamic vinegar

Directions:

1. Mix all ingredients.

Nutrition:

- Calories: 406
- Protein: 9g
- Carbohydrate: 32g
- Fat: 5g

44. Wild Rice Prawn Salad

Preparation Time: 5 Minutes
Cooking Time: 35 Minutes
Servings: 6
Ingredients:

- ¾ Cup wild rice
- 1¾ Cups chicken stock
- 1 Pound prawns
- Salt and pepper to taste
- 2 Tablespoons lemon juice
- 2 Tablespoons extra virgin olive oil
- 2 Cups arugula

Directions:

1. Combine the rice and chicken stock in a saucepan and cook until the liquid has been absorbed entirely.
2. Transfer the rice to a salad bowl.
3. Season the prawns with salt and pepper and drizzle them with lemon juice and oil.
4. Heat a grill pan over a medium flame.
5. Place the prawns on the hot pan and cook on each side for 2-3 minutes.
6. For the salad, combine the rice with arugula and prawns and mix well.
7. Serve the salad fresh.

Nutrition:

- Calories: 207
- Fat: 4g
- Protein: 20.6g
- Carbohydrates: 17g

45. Beet Salad (from Israel)

Preparation Time: 5 Minutes
Cooking Time: 0 Minutes
Servings: 2
Ingredients:

- 2–3 Fresh, raw beets grated or shredded in food processor
- 3 Tablespoons olive oil
- 2 Tablespoons balsamic vinegar
- ¼ Teaspoon salt
- 1/3 Teaspoon cumin
- Dash stevia powder or liquid
- Dash pepper

Directions:

1. Mix all ingredients together for the best raw beet salad.

Nutrition:

- Calories: 156
- Protein: 8g
- Carbohydrate: 40g
- Fat: 5g

46. Greek Salad

Preparation Time: 15 Minutes
Cooking Time: 15 Minutes
Servings: 5
Ingredients:
For the Dressing:

- ½ Teaspoon black pepper
- ¼ Teaspoon salt
- ½ Teaspoon oregano
- 1 Tablespoon garlic powder
- 2 Tablespoons Balsamic
- 1/3 Cup olive oil

For the Salad:

- ½ Cup sliced black olives
- ½ Cup chopped parsley, fresh
- 1 Small red onion, thin-sliced
- 1 Cup cherry tomatoes, sliced
- 1 Bell pepper, yellow, chunked
- 1 Cucumber, peeled, quartered, and sliced
- 4 Cups chopped romaine lettuce
- ½ Teaspoon salt
- 2 Tablespoons olive oil

Directions:

1. In a small bowl, blend all of the ingredients for the dressing and let this set in the refrigerator while you make the salad.
2. To assemble the salad, mix together all the ingredients in a large-sized bowl and toss the veggies gently but thoroughly to mix.
3. Serve the salad with the dressing in amounts as desired

Nutrition:

- Calories: 234
- Fat: 16.1g
- Protein: 5g
- Carbs: 48g

47. Norwegian Niçoise Salad Smoked Salmon Cucumber Egg and Asparagus

Preparation Time: 20 Minutes
Cooking Time: 5 Minutes
Servings: 4
Ingredients:
For the vinaigrette:

- 3 Tablespoons walnut oil
- 2 Tablespoons champagne vinegar
- 1 Tablespoon chopped fresh dill
- ½ Teaspoon kosher salt
- ¼ Teaspoon ground mustard
- Freshly ground black pepper

For the salad:

- Handful green beans, trimmed
- 1 (3- to 4-ounce) Package spring greens
- 12 Spears pickled asparagus
- 4 Large soft-boiled eggs, halved
- 8 Ounces smoked salmon, thinly sliced
- 1 Cucumber, thinly sliced
- 1 Lemon, quartered

Directions:

1. To make the dressing. In a small bowl, whisk the oil, vinegar, dill, salt, ground mustard, and a few grinds of pepper until emulsified. Set aside.
2. To make the salad. Start by blanching the green beans, bring a pot of salted water to a boil. Drop in the beans. Cook for 1 to 2 minutes until they turn bright green, then immediately drain and rinse under cold water. Set aside.
3. Divide the spring greens among four plates. Toss each serving with dressing to taste. Arrange three asparagus spears, one egg, 2 ounces of salmon, one-fourth of the cucumber slices, and a lemon wedge on each plate. Serve immediately.

Nutrition:

- Calories: 257
- Total fat: 18g
- Total carbs: 6g
- Cholesterol: 199mg
- Fiber: 2g
- Protein: 19g
- Sodium: 603mg

48. Mediterranean Chickpea Salad

Preparation Time: 5 Minutes
Cooking Time: 20 Minutes
Servings: 6
Ingredients:

- 1 Can chickpeas, drained
- 1 Fennel bulb, sliced
- 1 Red onion, sliced
- 1 Teaspoon dried basil
- 1 Teaspoon dried oregano
- 2 Tablespoons chopped parsley
- 4 Garlic cloves, minced
- 2 Tablespoons lemon juice
- 2 Tablespoons extra virgin olive oil
- Salt and pepper to taste

Directions:

1. Combine the chickpeas, fennel, red onion, herbs, garlic, lemon juice, and oil in a salad bowl.
2. Add salt and pepper and serve the salad fresh.

Nutrition:

- Calories: 200
- Fat: 9g
- Protein: 4g
- Carbohydrates: 28g

49. Romaine Lettuce and Radicchios Mix

Preparation Time: 6 Minutes
Cooking Time: 0 Minutes
Servings: 4
Ingredients:

- 2 Tablespoons olive oil
- A pinch of salt and black pepper
- 2 Spring onions, chopped
- 3 Tablespoons Dijon mustard
- Juice of 1 lime
- ½ Cup basil, chopped
- 4 Cups romaine lettuce heads, chopped
- 3 Radicchios, sliced

Directions:

1. In a salad bowl, mix the lettuce with the spring onions and the other ingredients, toss and serve.

Nutrition:

- Calories: 87
- Fats: 2g
- Fiber: 1g
- Carbs: 1g
- Protein: 2g

50. Chicken Broccoli Salad With Avocado Dressing

Preparation Time: 5 Minutes
Cooking Time: 40 Minutes
Servings: 6
Ingredients:

- 2 Chicken breasts
- 1 Pound broccoli, cut into florets
- 1 Avocado, peeled and pitted
- ½ Lemon, juiced
- 2 Garlic cloves
- ¼ Teaspoon chili powder
- ¼ Teaspoon cumin powder
- Salt and pepper to taste

Directions:

1. Cook the chicken in a large pot of salty water.
2. Drain and cut the chicken into small cubes—place in a salad bowl.
3. Add the broccoli and mix well.
4. Combine the avocado, lemon juice, garlic, chili powder, cumin powder, salt, and pepper in a blender. Pulse until smooth.
5. Spoon the dressing over the salad and mix well.
6. Serve the salad fresh.

Nutrition:

- Calories: 195
- Fat: 11g
- Protein: 14g
- Carbohydrates: 3g

51. Zucchini Salmon Salad

Preparation Time: 5 Minutes
Cooking Time: 10 Minutes
Servings: 3
Ingredients:

- 2 Salmon fillets
- 2 Tablespoons soy sauce
- 2 Zucchinis, sliced
- Salt and pepper to taste
- 2 Tablespoons extra virgin olive oil
- 2 Tablespoons sesame seeds

Directions:

1. Drizzle the salmon with soy sauce.
2. Heat a grill pan over a medium flame. Cook salmon on the grill on each side for 2-3 minutes.
3. Season the zucchini with salt and pepper and place it on the grill as well. Cook on each side until golden.
4. Place the zucchini, salmon, and the rest of the ingredients in a bowl.
5. Serve the salad fresh.

Nutrition:

- Calories: 224
- Fat: 19g
- Protein: 18g
- Carbohydrates: 0g

52. Warm Chorizo Chickpea Salad

Preparation Time: 5 Minutes
Cooking Time: 20 Minutes
Servings: 6
Ingredients:

- 1 Tablespoon extra-virgin olive oil
- 4 Chorizo links, sliced
- 1 Red onion, sliced
- 4 Roasted red bell peppers, chopped
- 1 Can chickpeas, drained
- 2 Cups cherry tomatoes
- 2 Tablespoons balsamic vinegar
- Salt and pepper to taste

Directions:

1. Heat the oil in a skillet and add the chorizo. Cook briefly just until fragrant, then add the onion, bell peppers, and chickpeas and cook for two additional minutes.
2. Transfer the mixture to a salad bowl, then add the tomatoes, vinegar, salt, and pepper.
3. Mix well and serve the salad right away.

Nutrition:

- Calories: 359
- Fat: 18g
- Protein: 15g
- Carbohydrates: 21g

53. Broccoli Salad

Preparation Time: 5 Minutes
Cooking Time: 0 Minutes
Servings: 2
Ingredients:

- 1 Head broccoli, chopped
- 2–3 Slices of fried bacon, crumbled
- 1 Diced green onion
- ½ Cup raisins or craisins
- ½–1 Cup of chopped pecans
- ¾ Cups sunflower seeds
- ½ Cup of pomegranate

Dressing:

- 1 Cup Organic Mayonnaise
- ¼ Cup Baking Stevia
- 2 Teaspoons White Vinegar

Directions:

1. Mix all ingredients together. Mix dressing and fold into the salad.

Nutrition:

- Calories: 239
- Protein: 10g
- Carbohydrate: 33g
  Fat: 2g

Chapter 5. Soup and Stew Recipes

54. Roasted Tomato Soup

Difficulty: Easy
Preparation Time: 20 Minutes
Cooking Time: 50 Minutes
Servings: 6
Ingredients:

- 3 Pounds of tomatoes, halved (1green)
- 6 Garlic(smashed) (½ condiment)
- 4 Teaspoons of cooking oil or virgin oil (1/8 condiment)
- Salt to taste (1/8 condiment)
- 1/4 Cup of heavy cream (optional) (½ healthy fat)
- Sliced fresh basil leaves for garnish (1/8green)

Directions:

1. Set the oven at medium heat of about 427°F and let it preheat
2. In your mixing bowl, mix the halved tomatoes, garlic, olive oil, salt, and pepper
3. Spread the tomato mixture on the already prepared baking sheet
4. For a process of 20- 28 minutes, roast and stir
5. Then remove it from the oven, and the roasted vegetables should now be transferred to a soup pot
6. Stir in the basil leaves
7. Blend in small portions in a blender
8. Serve immediately

Nutrition:

- Fat: 5.9g
- Protein: 2.3g
- Calories: 126

55. Lemon-Garlic Chicken

Difficulty: Average
Preparation Time: 5 Minutes
Cooking Time: 45 Minutes
Servings: 4
Ingredients:

- 1 Small lemon, juiced (1/8 condiment)
- 1 3/4 lb. of bone-in, skinless chicken thighs (1 lean)
- 2 Tablespoons of fresh oregano, minced (1/8green)
- 2 Cloves of garlic, minced (1/8 condiment)
- 2 lbs. of asparagus, trimmed (1/8green)
- 1/4 Teaspoon each or less for black pepper and salt (1/8 condiment)

Directions:

1. Preheat the oven to about 350°F. Put the chicken in a medium-sized bowl.
2. Now, add the garlic, oregano, lemon juice, pepper, and salt and toss together to combine.
3. Roast for 40 minutes.
4. Once the chicken thighs have been cooked, remove and keep them aside to rest.
5. Now, steam the asparagus on a stovetop or in a microwave to the desired doneness.
6. Serve asparagus with roasted chicken thighs.

Nutrition:

- Calories: 350
- Fat: 10g
- Protein: 32g

56. Quick Lentil Chili

Difficulty: Easy
Preparation Time: 15 Minutes
Cooking Time: 1 Hour and 20 Minutes
Servings: 10
Ingredients:

- 1½ Cups of seeded or diced pepper (1green)
  5 Cups of vegetable broth (it should have a low sodium
- content) (1 condiment)
- 1 Tablespoon of garlic (1/8 condiment)
- 1/4 Teaspoon of freshly ground pepper (1/8 condiment)
- 1 Cup of red lentils (1/4green)
- 3 Filled teaspoons of chili powder (1/8 condiment)
- 1 Tablespoon of grounded cumin (1/8 condiment)

Directions:

1. Place your pot over medium heat
2. Combine your onions, red peppers, low sodium vegetable broth, garlic, salt, and pepper
3. Cook and always stir until the onions are more translucent and all the liquid evaporated. This will take about 10mins.
4. Add the remaining broth, lime juice, chili powder, lentils, cumin, and boil.
5. Reduce heat at this point, cover it for about 15 minutes to simmer until the lentils are appropriately cooked
6. Drizzle a little water if the mixture seems to be thick.
7. The chili will be appropriately done when most of the water is absorbed.
8. Serve and enjoy.

Nutrition:

- Protein: 2.3g
- Calories: 121
- Fat: 2.9g

57. Creamy Cauliflower Soup

Difficulty: Average
Preparation Time: 15 Minutes
Cooking Time: 30 Minutes
Servings: 6
Ingredients:

- 5 Cups cauliflower rice (1green)
- 8 oz. Cheddar cheese, grated (1 healthy fat)
- 2 Cups unsweetened almond milk (½ healthy fat)
- 2 Cups vegetable stock (1 condiment)
- 2 Tbsp. water (½ condiment)
- 2 Garlic cloves, minced (1/4 condiment)
- 1 Tbsp. olive oil (1/8 condiment)

Directions:

1. Cook olive oil in a large stockpot over medium heat.
2. Add garlic and cook for 1-2 minutes. Add cauliflower rice and water.
3. Cover and cook for 5-7 minutes.
4. Now add vegetable stock and almond milk and stir well.
5. Bring to a boil.
6. Turn heat to low and simmer for 5 minutes.
7. Turn off the heat.
8. Slowly add cheddar cheese and stir until smooth.
9. Season soup with pepper and salt.
10. Stir well and serve hot.

Nutrition:

- Calories: 214
- Fat: 16.5g
- Protein: 11.6g

58. Crackpot Chicken Taco Soup

Difficulty: Average
Preparation Time: 15 Minutes
Cooking Time: 6 Hours
Servings: 6
Ingredients:

- 2 Frozen boneless chicken breasts (1 lean)
- 2 Cans of white beans or black beans (1 healthy fat)
- 1 Can of diced tomatoes (1 healthy fat)
- ½ Packet of taco seasoning (1/8 condiment)
- ½ Teaspoon of Garlic salt (1/8 condiment)
- 1 Cup of chicken broth (1 condiment)
- Salt and pepper to taste (1/8 condiment)
- Tortilla chips, sour cream cheese, and cilantro as toppings (1 healthy fat)

Directions:

1. Put your frozen chicken into the crockpot and place the other ingredients into the pool too.
2. Leave to cook for about 6-8 hours.
3. After cooking, take out the chicken and shred it to the size you want.
4. Finally, place the shredded chicken into the crockpot and put it on a slow cooker. Stir and allow to cook.
5. You can add more beans and tomatoes also to help stretch the meat and make it tastier.

Nutrition:

- Protein: 29g
- Fat: 4g
- Calories: 171

59. Cheeseburger Soup

Difficulty: Average
Preparation Time: 15 Minutes
Cooking Time: 45 Minutes
Servings: 4
Ingredients:

- 1 14.5 oz. can diced tomato (1green)
- 1 lb. of 90% lean ground beef (1 lean)
- 3/4 Cup of chopped celery (½ green)
- 2 Teaspoons of Worcestershire sauce (1/8 condiment)
- 3 Cups of low sodium chicken broth (1 condiment)
- 1/4 Teaspoon of salt (1/8 condiment)
- 1 Teaspoon of dried parsley (1/8green)
- 7 Cups of baby spinach (1green)
- 1/4 Teaspoon of ground pepper (1/8 condiment)
- 4 oz. of reduced-fat shredded cheddar cheese (½ healthy fat)

Directions:

1. Get a large soup pot and cook the beef until it becomes brown.
2. Add the celery and sauté until it becomes tender.
3. Remove from the heat and drain excess liquid. Stir in the broth, tomatoes, parsley, Worcestershire sauce, pepper, and salt.
4. Cover with the lid and allow it to simmer on low heat for about 20 minutes.
5. Add spinach and leave it to cook until it becomes wilted in about 1-3 minutes.
6. Top each of your servings with 1 ounce of cheese.

Nutrition:

- Calories: 400
- Protein: 44g
- Fat: 20g

60. Mushroom & Jalapeño Stew

Difficulty: Easy
Preparation Time: 20 Minutes
Cooking Time: 50 Minutes
Servings: 4
Ingredients:

- 2 Tsp. olive oil (1/8 condiment)
- 1 Cup leeks, chopped (½ green)
- 1 Garlic clove, minced (1/8 condiment)
- ½ Cup celery stalks, chopped (½ green)
- ½ Cup carrots, chopped (½ green)
- 1 Green bell pepper, chopped (½ green)
- 1 Jalapeño pepper, chopped (1/4green)
- 2 ½ Cups mushrooms, sliced (1 healthy fat)
- 1 ½ Cups vegetable stock (1 condiment)
- 2 Tomatoes, chopped (1green)
- 2 Thyme sprigs, chopped (1/4green)
- 1 Rosemary sprig, chopped (1/4green)
- 2 Bay leaves (1/4green)
- ½ Tsp. salt (1/8 condiment)
- 1/4 Tsp. ground black pepper (1/8 condiment)
- 2 Tbsp. vinegar (1/8 condiment)

Directions:

1. Set a pot over medium heat and warm oil.
2. Add in garlic and leeks and sauté until soft and translucent.
3. Add in the black pepper, celery, mushrooms, and carrots.
4. Cook as you stir for 12 minutes; stir in a splash of vegetable stock to ensure there is no sticking.
5. Stir in the rest of the ingredients.
6. Set heat to medium; allow to simmer for 25 to 35 minutes or until cooked through.
7. Divide into individual bowls and serve warm.

Nutrition:

- Calories: 65
- Fats: 2.7g
- Protein: 2.7g

61. Easy Cauliflower Soup

Difficulty: Easy
Preparation Time: 5 Minutes
Cooking Time: 15 Minutes
Servings: 4
Ingredients:

- 2 Tbsp. olive oil (1/4 condiment)
- 1 Tsp. garlic, minced (1/4 condiment)
- 1-pound cauliflower, cut into florets (1green)
- 1 Cup kale, chopped (½ green)
- 4 Cups vegetable broth (1 condiment)
- ½ Cup almond milk (½ healthy fat)
- ½ Tsp. salt (1/8 condiment)
- ½ Tsp. red pepper flakes (1/8 condiment)
- 1 Tbsp. fresh chopped parsley (1/4green)

Directions:

1. Set a pot over medium heat and warm the oil.
2. Add garlic and onions and sauté until browned and softened.
3. Place in vegetable broth, kale, and cauliflower; cook for 10 minutes until the mixture boils.
4. Stir in the pepper flakes, salt, and almond milk; reduce the heat and simmer the soup for 5 minutes.
5. Transfer the soup to an immersion blender and blend to achieve the desired consistency; top with parsley and serve immediately.

Nutrition:

- Calories: 172
- Fats: 10.3g
- Protein: 8.1g

62. Tofu Stir Fry With Asparagus Stew

Difficulty: Average
Preparation Time: 15 Minutes
Cooking Time: 30 Minutes
Servings: 4
Ingredients:

- 1-pound Asparagus, cut off stems (1green)
- 2 Tbsp. olive oil (1/8 condiment)
- 2 Blocks tofu, pressed and cubed (1 lean)
- 2 Garlic cloves, minced (1/8 condiment)
- 1 Tsp. Cajun spice mix (1/8 condiment)
- 1 Tsp. mustard (1/8 condiment)
- 1 Bell pepper, chopped (1/4green)
- 1/4 Cup vegetable broth (1green)
- Salt and black pepper, to taste (1/8 condiment)

Directions:

1. Using a huge saucepan with lightly salted water, place in asparagus and cook until tender for 10 minutes; drain.
2. Set a wok over high heat and warm olive oil; stir in tofu cubes and cook for 6 minutes.
3. Place in garlic and cook for 30 seconds until soft.
4. Stir in the remaining ingredients, including reserved asparagus, and cook for four more minutes.
5. Divide among plates and serve.

Nutrition:

- Calories: 138
- Fat: 8.9g
- Protein: 6.4g

63. Cream of Thyme Tomato Soup

Difficulty: Easy
Preparation Time: 5 Minutes
Cooking Time: 20 Minutes
Servings: 6
Ingredients:

- 2 Tbsp. ghee (½ healthy fat)
- ½ Cup raw cashew nuts, diced (½ healthy fat)
- 2 (28 oz.) Cans tomatoes (1green)
- 1 Tsp. fresh thyme leaves + extra to garnish (1/4green)
- 1 ½ Cups water (½ healthy fat)
- Salt and black pepper to taste (1/8 condiment)

Directions:

1. Cook ghee in a pot over medium heat and sauté the onions for 4 minutes until softened.
2. Stir in the tomatoes, thyme, water, cashews, and season with salt and black pepper.
3. Cover and bring to simmer for 10 minutes until thoroughly cooked.
4. Open, turn the heat off, and puree the ingredients with an immersion blender.
5. Adjust to taste and stir in the heavy cream.
6. Spoon into soup bowls and serve.

Nutrition:

- Calories: 310
- Fats: 27g
- Protein: 11g

64. Lime-Mint Soup

Difficulty: Difficult
Preparation Time: 5 Minutes
Cooking Time: 20 Minutes
Servings: 4
Ingredients:

- 4 Cups vegetable broth (1 condiment)
- 1/4 Cup fresh mint leaves (1/8 condiment)
- 1/4 Cup scallions (1/4green)
- 3 Garlic cloves, minced (1/8 condiment)
- 3 Tablespoons freshly squeezed lime juice (1/4 condiment)

Directions:

1. In a large stockpot, combine the broth, mint, scallions, garlic, and lime juice.
2. Bring to a boil over medium-high heat.
3. Cover, set heat to low, simmer for 15 minutes, and serve.

Nutrition:

- Fat: 2g
- Protein: 5g
- Calories: 214

Chapter 6. Vegan Recipes

65. Vegan Edamame Quinoa Collard Wraps

Preparation Time: 5 Minutes
Cooking Time: 15 Minutes
Servings: 4
Ingredients:
For the wrap:

- 2 to 3 Collard leaves
- 1/4 Cup Grated carrot
- 1/4 Cup Sliced cucumber
- 1/4 Thin strips Red bell pepper
- 1/4 Thin strips Orange bell pepper
- 1/3 Cup Cooked Quinoa
- 1/3 Cup Shelled defrosted edamame

For the dressing:

- 3 Tablespoons Fresh ginger root, peeled and chopped
- 1 Cup Cooked chickpeas
- 1 Garlic clove
- 4 Tablespoons Rice vinegar
- 2 Tablespoons Low sodium tamari/coconut aminos
- 2 Tablespoons Lime juice
- 1/4 Cup Water
- Few pinches of chili flakes
- 1 Stevia pack

Directions:

1. For the dressing, combine all the ingredients and purée in a food processor until smooth.
2. Load into a little jar or tub, and set aside.
3. Place the collar leaves on a flat surface, covering one another to create a tighter tie.
4. Take one tablespoon of ginger dressing and blend it up with the prepared quinoa.
5. Spoon the prepared quinoa onto the leaves and shape a simple horizontal line at the closest end.
6. Supplement the edamame with all the veggie fillings left over.
7. Drizzle around one tablespoon of the ginger dressing on top, then fold the cover's sides inwards.
8. Pullover the fillings, the side of the cover closest to you, then turn the whole body away to seal it up.

Nutrition:

- Calories: 295
- Sugar: 3g
- Sodium: 200mg
- Fat: 13g

66. Baked Cheesy Eggplant With Marinara

Preparation Time: 20 Minutes
Cooking Time: 45 Minutes
Servings: 3
Ingredients:

- 1 Clove garlic, sliced
- 1 Large eggplant
- 2 Tablespoons olive oil
- ½ Pinch salt, or as needed
- 1/4 Cup and 2 tablespoons dry bread crumbs
- 1/4 Cup and 2 tablespoons ricotta cheese
- 1/4 Cup grated Parmesan cheese
- 1/4 Cup water, plus more as needed
- 1/4 Teaspoon red pepper flakes
- 1-½ Cups prepared marinara sauce
- 1-½ Teaspoons olive oil
- 2 Tablespoons shredded pepper jack cheese
- Salt and freshly ground black pepper to taste

Directions:

1. Cut the eggplant crosswise into five pieces. Peel a pumpkin, grate it and cut it into two cubes.

2. Lightly turn skillet with one tablespoon olive oil. Heat the oil at 390°F for 5 minutes. Add half of the eggplants and cook for 2 minutes on each side. Transfer to a plate.
3. Add one tablespoon of olive oil and add garlic, cook for one minute. Add the chopped eggplants. Season with pepper flakes and salt. Cook for 4 minutes. Lower the heat to 330oF and continue cooking the eggplants until soft, about eight more minutes.
4. Stir in water and marinara sauce. Cook for 7 minutes until heated through. Stir every now and then. Transfer to a bowl.
5. In a bowl, whisk well pepper, salt, pepper jack cheese, Parmesan cheese, and ricotta. Evenly spread cheeses over eggplant strips and then fold in half.
6. Lay folded eggplant in baking pan. Pour the marinara sauce on top.
7. In a small bowl, whisk well olive oil and bread crumbs. Sprinkle all over the sauce.
8. Cook for 15 minutes at 390°F until tops are lightly browned.
9. Serve and enjoy.

Nutrition:

- Calories: 405
- Carbs: 41.1g
- Protein: 12.7g
- Fat: 21.4g

67. Creamy Spinach and Mushroom Lasagna

Preparation Time: 60 Minutes
Cooking Time: 20 Minutes
Servings: 6
Ingredients:

- 10 Lasagna noodles
- 1 Package whole milk ricotta
- 2 Packages of frozen chopped spinach.
- 4 Cups mozzarella cheese (divided and shredded)
- 3/4 Cups grated fresh Parmesan
- 3 Tablespoons chopped fresh parsley leaves (optional)

For the Sauce:

- 1/4 Cup of butter (unsalted)
- 2 Garlic cloves
- 1 Pound of thinly sliced cremini mushroom
- 1 Diced onion
- 1/4 Cup flour
- 4 Cups milk, kept at room temperature
- 1 Teaspoon basil (dried)
- Pinch of nutmeg
- Salt and freshly ground black pepper, to taste

Directions:

1. Preheat oven to 352 degrees F.
2. To make the sauce, over medium heat, melt your butter. Add garlic, mushrooms, and onion. Cook and stir at intervals until it becomes tender at about 3-4 minutes.
3. Whisk in flour until lightly browned; it takes about 1 minute for it to become brown.
4. Next, whisk in the milk gradually, and cook, constantly whisking, about 2-3 minutes till it becomes thickened. Stir in basil, oregano, and nutmeg, season with salt and pepper for taste.
5. Then set aside.
6. In another pot of boiling salted water, cook lasagna noodles according to the package instructions.
7. Spread one cup mushroom sauce onto the bottom of a baking dish; top it with four lasagna noodles, ½ of the spinach, one cup mozzarella cheese, and 1/4 cup Parmesan.
8. Repeat this process with the remaining noodles, mushroom sauce, and cheeses.

9. Place into oven and bake for 35-45 minutes, or until it starts bubbling. Then boil for 2-3 minutes until it becomes brown and translucent.
10. Let cool for 15 minutes.
11. Serve it with garnished parsley (optional)

Nutrition:

- Calories: 488.3 Cal
- Fats: 19.3g
- Cholesterol: 88.4mg
- Sodium: 451.9mg
- Carbohydrates: 51.0g
- Dietary Fiber: 7.0g
- Protein: 25.0g

68. Zucchini Parmesan Chips

Difficulty: Hard
Preparation Time: 5 Minutes
Cooking Time: 8 Minutes
Servings: 10
Ingredients:

- ½ Tsp. Paprika
- ½ C. Grated parmesan cheese
- ½ C. Italian breadcrumbs
- 1 Lightly beaten egg
- Thinly sliced zucchinis

Directions:

1. Use a very sharp knife or mandolin slicer to slice zucchini as thinly as you can—pat off extra moisture.
2. Beat the egg with a pinch of pepper and salt and a bit of water.
3. Combine paprika, cheese, and breadcrumbs in a bowl.
4. Dip slices of zucchini into the egg mixture and then into the breadcrumb mixture. Press gently to coat.
5. With olive oil or cooking spray, mist-coated zucchini slices, then place them into your air fryer in a single layer.
6. Cook 8 minutes at 350 degrees.
7. Sprinkle with salt and serve with salsa.

Nutrition:

- Calories: 211
- Fat: 16g
- Protein: 8g
- Sugar: 0g

69. Roasted Squash Puree

Preparation Time: 20 Minutes
Cooking Time: 6 to 7 Hours
Servings: 8
Ingredients:

- 1 (3-pound) Butternut squash, peeled, seeded, and cut into 1-inch pieces
- 3 (1-pound) Acorn squash, peeled, seeded, and cut into 1-inch pieces
- 2 Onions, chopped
- 3 Garlic cloves, minced
- 2 Tablespoons olive oil
- 1 Teaspoon dried marjoram leaves
- ½ Teaspoon salt
- 1/8 Teaspoon freshly ground black pepper

Directions:

1. In a 6-quart slow cooker, mix all of the ingredients.
2. Cover and cook on low for 6 to 7 hours or until the squash is tender when pierced with a fork.
3. Use a potato masher to mash the squash right in the slow cooker.

Nutrition:

- Calories: 175
- Carbohydrates: 38g
- Sugar: 1g
- Fiber: 3g
- Fat: 4g
- Saturated Fat: 1g
- Protein: 3g
- Sodium: 149mg

70. Air Fryer Brussels Sprouts

Difficulty: Hard
Preparation Time: 5 Minutes
Cooking Time: 10 Minutes
Servings: 5
Ingredients:

- ¼ Tsp. salt
- 1 Tbsp. balsamic vinegar
- 1 Tbsp. olive oil
- C. Brussels sprouts

Directions:

1. Cut Brussels sprouts in half lengthwise. Toss with salt, vinegar, and olive oil till coated thoroughly.
2. Add coated sprouts to the air fryer, cooking 8-10 minutes at 400 degrees. Shake after 5 minutes of cooking.
3. Brussels sprouts are ready to devour when brown and crisp!

Nutrition:

- Calories: 118
- Fat: 9g
- Protein: 11g
- Sugar: 1g

71. Thai Roasted Veggies

Preparation Time: 20 Minutes
Cooking Time: 6 to 8 Hours
Servings: 8
Ingredients:

- 4 Large carrots, peeled and cut into chunks
- 2 Onions, peeled and sliced
- 6 Garlic cloves, peeled and sliced
- 2 Parsnips, peeled and sliced
- 2 Jalapeño peppers, minced
- ½ Cup Roasted Vegetable Broth
- 1/3 Cup canned coconut milk
- 3 Tablespoons lime juice
- 2 Tablespoons grated fresh ginger root
- 2 Teaspoons curry powder

Directions:

1. In a 6-quart slow cooker, mix the carrots, onions, garlic, parsnips, and jalapeño peppers.
2. In a small bowl, mix the vegetable broth, coconut milk, lime juice, ginger root, and curry powder until well blended. Pour this mixture into the slow cooker.
3. Cover and cook on low for 6 to 8 hours, do it until the vegetables are tender when pierced with a fork.

Nutrition:

- Calories: 69
- Carbohydrates: 13g
- Sugar: 6g
- Fiber: 3g
- Fat: 3g
- Saturated Fat: 3g
- Protein: 1g
- Sodium: 95mg

72. Crispy Jalapeno Coins

Difficulty: Hard
Preparation Time: 10 Minutes
Cooking Time: 10 Minutes
Servings: 8 to 10
Ingredients:

- 1 Egg
- 2-3 Tbsp. coconut flour
- 1 Sliced and seeded jalapeno
- Pinch of garlic powder
- Pinch of onion powder
- Pinch of Cajun seasoning (optional)
- Pinch of pepper and salt

Directions:

1. Ensure your air fryer is preheated to 400 degrees.
2. Mix together all dry ingredients.
3. Pat jalapeno slices dry. Dip coins into the egg wash and then into the dry mixture. Toss to thoroughly coat.
4. Add coated jalapeno slices to the air fryer in a singular layer. Spray with olive oil.
5. Cook just till crispy.

Nutrition:

- Calories: 128
- Fat: 8g
- Protein: 7g
- Sugar: 0g

73. Crispy-Topped Baked Vegetables

Preparation Time: 10 Minutes
Cooking Time: 40 Minutes
Servings: 4
Ingredients:

- 2 Tbsp. Olive oil
- 1 Onion, chopped
- 1 Celery stalk, chopped
- 2 Carrots, grated
- ½-pound Turnips, sliced
- 1 Cup vegetable broth
- 1 Tsp. Turmeric
- Sea salt and black pepper, to taste
- ½ Tsp. Liquid smoke
- 1 Cup Parmesan cheese, shredded
- 2 Tbsp. Fresh chives, chopped

Directions:

1. Set oven to 360ºF and grease a baking dish with olive oil.
2. Set a skillet over medium heat and warm olive oil.
3. Sweat the onion until soft, and place in the turnips, carrots, and celery; and cook for 4 minutes.
4. Remove the vegetable mixture from the baking dish.
5. Combine vegetable broth with turmeric, pepper, liquid smoke, and salt.
6. Spread this mixture over the vegetables.
7. Sprinkle with Parmesan cheese and bake for about 30 minutes.
8. Garnish with chives to serve.

Nutrition:

- Calories: 242 Cal
- Fats: 16.3g
- Carbohydrates: 8.6g
- Protein: 16.3g

74. Jicama Fries

Difficulty: Hard
Preparation Time: 10 Minutes
Cooking Time: 20 Minutes
Servings: 8
Ingredients:

- 1 Tbsp. Dried thyme
- ¾ C. Arrowroot flour
- ½ Large Jicama
- Eggs

Directions:

1. Sliced jicama into fries.
2. Whisk eggs together and pour over fries. Toss to coat.
3. Mix a pinch of salt, thyme, and arrowroot flour together. Toss egg-coated jicama into dry mixture, tossing to coat well.
4. Spray air fryer basket with olive oil and add fries—cook 20 minutes on the "CHIPS" setting. Toss halfway into the cooking process.

Nutrition:

- Calories: 211
- Fat: 19g
- Protein: 9g
- Sugar: 1g

75. Spaghetti Squash Tots

Difficulty: Hard
Preparation Time: 5 Minutes
Cooking Time: 15 Minutes
Servings: 8 to 10
Ingredients:

- ¼ Tsp. pepper
- ½ Tsp. salt
- 1 Thinly sliced scallion
- 1 Spaghetti squash

Directions:

1. Wash and cut the squash in half lengthwise. Scrap out the seeds.
2. With a fork, remove spaghetti meat by strands and throw out skins.
3. In a clean towel, toss in squash and wring out as much moisture as possible. Place in a bowl and with a knife, slice through meat a few times to cut up smaller.
4. Add pepper, salt, and scallions to squash and mix well.
5. Create "tot" shapes with your hands and place them in the air fryer. Spray with olive oil.
6. Cook 15 minutes at 350 degrees until golden and crispy!

Nutrition:

- Calories: 231
- Fat: 18g
- Protein: 5g
- Sugar: 0g

76. Low Carb Pork Dumplings With Dipping Sauce

Difficulty: Difficult
Preparation Time: 30 Minutes
Cooking Time: 20 Minutes
Servings: 6
Ingredients:

- 18 Dumpling wrappers (1 healthy fat)
- 1 Teaspoon olive oil (1/4 condiment)
- 4 Cups bok choy (chopped) (2 leans)
- 2 Tablespoons rice vinegar (½ condiment)
- 1 Tablespoon diced ginger (1/4 condiment)
- 1/4 Teaspoon crushed red pepper (½ green)
- 1 Tablespoon diced garlic (½ condiment)
- Lean ground pork ½ cup (2 leans)
- 2 Teaspoons Lite soy sauce (½ condiment)
- ½ Tsp. Honey (1/4 healthy fat)
- 1 Teaspoon Toasted sesame oil (1/4 condiment)
- Finely chopped scallions (1green)

Directions

1. In a large skillet, heat the olive oil, add the bok choy, cook for 6 minutes and add the garlic, ginger and cook for one minute. Transfer this mixture to a paper towel and pat dry any excess oil
2. In a bowl, add the mixture of bok choy, red pepper, and lean ground pork and mix well.
3. Place dumplings wrap on a plate and add a spoon to fill half of the wrapper. With water, seal the edges and fold them.
4. Spray air fryer basket with oil, add dumplings into the air fryer basket and cook at 375°F for 12 minutes or until golden brown.
5. Meanwhile, to make the sauce, combine the sesame oil, rice vinegar, shallot, soy sauce, and honey in a mixing bowl.
6. Serve the dumplings with the sauce.

Nutrition:

- Calories: 140
- Fat: 5g
- Protein: 12g

77. Gluten-Free Air Fryer Chicken Fried Brown Rice

Difficulty: Average
Preparation Time: 10 Minutes
Cooking Time: 20 Minutes
Servings: 2
Ingredients:

- 1 Cup Chicken Breast (1 lean)
- 1/4 Cup chopped White Onion (½ green)
- 1/4 Cup chopped Celery (½ green)
- 4 Cups Cooked brown rice (2 healthy fat)
- 1/4 Cup chopped Carrots (½ green)

Directions

1. Place the foil on the air fryer basket, make sure to leave room for airflow, roll up on the sides
2. Spray the film with olive oil. Mix all the ingredients.
3. On top of the foil, add all the ingredients to the air fryer basket.
4. Give a splash of olive oil to the mixture.
5. Cook for five minutes at 390°F.
6. Open the air fryer and give the mixture a spin
7. Cook for another five minutes at 390°F.
8. Remove from the air fryer and serve hot.

Nutrition

- Calories: 350
- Fat: 6g
- Protein: 22g

78. Air Fryer Cheesy Pork Chops

Difficulty: Average
Preparation Time: 5 Minutes
Cooking Time: 8 Minutes
Servings: 2
Ingredients:

- 2 Lean pork chops
- Half teaspoon of Salt (1/4 condiment)
- ½ Tsp. Garlic powder (1/4 condiment)
- 4 Tbsp. Shredded cheese (1 healthy fat)
- Chopped cilantro (1green)

Directions:

1. Let the air fryer preheat to 350 degrees.
2. With garlic, coriander and salt, rub the pork chops. Put the air fryer on. Let it cook for four minutes. Turn them over and then cook for extra two minutes.
3. Drizzle the cheese on top and cook for another two minutes or until the cheese has melted.
4. Serve with salad.

Nutrition

- Calories: 467
- Protein: 61g
- Fat: 22g

79. Air Fryer Pork Chop & Broccoli

Difficulty: Average
Preparation Time: 20 Minutes
Cooking Time: 20 Minutes
Servings: 2
Ingredients:

- 2 Cups Broccoli florets (1green)
- 2 Pieces Bone-in pork chop (1 lean)
- ½ Tsp. Paprika (1/4 condiment)
- 2 Tbsp. Avocado oil (1 healthy fat)
- ½ Tsp. Garlic powder (1/4 condiment)
- ½ Tsp. Onion powder (1/4 condiment)
- Two cloves of crushed garlic (1/4 condiment)
- 1 Teaspoon of Salt divided (1/4 condiment)

Directions:

1. Let the air fryer preheat to 350 degrees. Spray the basket with cooking oil
2. Add an oil spoon, onion powder, half a teaspoon. of salt, garlic powder, and paprika in a bowl mix well, rub this spice mixture on the sides of the pork chop
3. Add the pork chops to the fryer basket and cook for five minutes
4. Meanwhile, add an oil teaspoon, garlic, a half teaspoon of salt, and broccoli in a bowl and coat them well
5. Turn the pork chop and add the broccoli, let it cook for another five minutes.
6. Remove from the air fryer and serve.

Nutrition:

- Calories: 483
- Fat: 20g
- Protein: 23g

80. Mustard Glazed Air Fryer Pork Tenderloin

Difficulty: Average
Preparation Time: 10 Minutes
Cooking Time: 18 Minutes
Servings: 4
Ingredients:

- ¼ Cup Yellow mustard (½ green)
- One pork tenderloin (1 lean)
- ¼ Tsp. Salt (1/4 condiment)
- 3 Tbsp. Honey (½ healthy fat)
- 1/8 Tsp. Black pepper (1/4 condiment)
- 1 Tbsp. Minced garlic (1/4 condiment)
- 1 Tsp. Dried rosemary (1/4green)
- 1 Tsp. Italian seasoning (1/8 condiment)

Directions:

1. Using a knife, cut the top of the pork tenderloin. Add the garlic (minced) into the cuts. Then sprinkle with kosher salt and pepper.
2. In a bowl, add the honey, mustard, rosemary, and Italian seasoning mixture until well blended. Rub this mustard mix all over the pork.
3. Leave to marinate in the refrigerator for at least two hours.
4. Place the pork tenderloin in the basket of the air fryer. Cook for 18-20 minutes at 400°F. With an instant-read thermometer, verify that the internal temperature of the pig should be 145°F.
5. Remove from the air fryer and serve with a side of salad.

Nutrition:

- Calories: 390
- Protein: 59g
- Fat: 11g

81. Air Fryer Pork Taquitos

Difficulty: Average
Preparation Time: 10 Minutes
Cooking Time: 20 Minutes
Servings: 10
Ingredients:

- 3 Cups of Pork tenderloin, cooked & shredded (2 leans)
- 2 and ½ cups, fat-free Shredded mozzarella (1 healthy fat)
- 10 Small tortillas (1 healthy fat)
- Salsa for dipping (1 condiment)
- Juice of a lime (1/4 condiment)

Directions:

1. Allow the air fryer to preheat to 380°F.
2. Add the lime juice to the pork and mix well
3. With a damp towel over the tortilla, microwave for ten seconds to soften it
4. Add the pork filling and cheese on top in a tortilla, roll the tortilla tightly.
5. Situate the tortillas on a greased baking sheet
6. Sprinkle oil on the tortillas. Bake for 7-10 minutes or until the tortillas are golden; turn them halfway.
7. Serve with salad.

Nutrition:

- Calories: 253
- Fat: 18g
- Protein: 20g

82. Pork Rind Nachos

Difficulty: Average
Preparation Time: 5 Minutes
Cooking Time: 5 Minutes
Servings: 2
Ingredients:

- Tbsp. Of pork rinds (1 lean)
- 1/4 Cup shredded cooked chicken (½ lean)
- ½ Cup shredded Monterey jack cheese (1/4 healthy fat)
- 1/4 Cup sliced pickled jalapeños (1/4green)
- 1/4 Cup guacamole (1/4 healthy fat)
- 1/4 Cup full-fat sour cream (1/4 healthy fat)

Directions:

1. Place the pork rinds in a 6-inch round pan. Fill with grilled chicken and Monterey jack cheese. Place the pan in the basket with the air fryer.
2. Set the temperature to 370°F and set the timer for 5 minutes or until the cheese has melted.
3. Eat immediately with jalapeños, guacamole, and sour cream.

Nutrition:

- Calories: 295
- Protein: 30g
- Fat: 27g

83. Air Fried Jamaican Jerk Pork

Difficulty: Difficult
Preparation Time: 10 Minutes
Cooking Time: 20 Minutes
Servings: 4
Ingredients:

- Pork, cut into three-inch pieces (1 lean)
- ¼ Cup Jerk paste (1/4 condiment)

Directions:

1. Rub the jerk dough on all the pork pieces.
2. Chill to marinate for 4 hours in the refrigerator.
3. Allow the air fryer to preheat to 390°F. Spray with olive oil
4. Before placing it in the air fryer, allow the meat to rest for 20 minutes at room temperature.
5. Cook for 20 minutes at 390°F in the air fryer, turn halfway.
6. Remove from the air fryer and let sit for ten minutes before slicing.
7. Serve with microgreens.

Nutrition:

- Calories: 234
- Protein: 31g
- Fat: 9g

84. Beef Lunch Meatballs

Difficulty: Easy
Preparation Time: 10 Minutes
Cooking Time: 15 Minutes
Servings: 4
Ingredients:

- ½ Pound beef, ground (½ lean)
- ½ Pound Italian sausage, chopped (½ lean)
- ½ Tsp. Garlic powder (1/4 condiment)
- ½ Tsp. Onion powder (1/4 condiment)
- Salt and black pepper to the taste (1/4 condiment)
- ½ Cup cheddar cheese, grated (½ healthy fat)
- Mashed potatoes for serving (½ healthy fat)

Directions:

1. In a bowl, mix the beef with the sausage, garlic powder, onion powder, salt, pepper, and cheese, mix well and form 16 meatballs with this mixture.

2. Place the meatballs in your air fryer and cook them at 370°F for 15 minutes.
3. Serve the meatballs with some mashed potatoes on the side.

Nutrition:

- Calories: 132
- Fat: 6.7g
- Protein: 5.5g

85. Air Fryer Whole Wheat Crusted Pork Chops

Difficulty: Average
Preparation Time: 10 Minutes
Cooking Time: 12 Minutes
Servings: 4
Ingredients:

- 1 Cup whole-wheat breadcrumbs (½ healthy fat)
- ¼ Teaspoon salt (1/4 condiment)
- 2-4 Pieces pork chops (center cut and boneless) (2 leans)
- ½ Teaspoon Chili powder (1/4 condiment)
- 1 Tablespoon parmesan cheese (1/4 healthy fat)
- 1 ½ Teaspoons paprika (½ condiment)
- 1 Egg beaten (1 healthy fat)
- ½ Teaspoon Onion powder (1/4 condiment)
- ½ Teaspoon Granulated garlic (1/4 condiment)

Directions:

1. Allow the air fryer to preheat to 400°F.
2. Rub kosher salt on each side of the pork chops, let them rest
3. Add the beaten egg to a large bowl
4. Add the parmesan, breadcrumbs, garlic, pepper, paprika, chili powder, and onion powder to a bowl and mix well
5. Dip the pork chop in the egg and then in the breadcrumbs
6. Put it in the air fryer and spray it with oil.
7. Leave them to cook for 12 minutes at 400°F. Turn them upside down halfway through cooking. Cook for another six minutes.
8. Serve with salad.

Nutrition:

- Calories: 425
- Fat: 20g
- Protein: 31g

86. Air Fried Philly Cheesesteak Taquitos

Difficulty: Average
Preparation Time: 20 Minutes
Cooking Time: 6-8 Hours
Servings: 6
Ingredients:

- 1 Package Dry Italian dressing mix (1 condiment)
- 1 Pack Super Soft Corn Tortillas (1 healthy fat)
- 2 Pieces green peppers chopped (½ green)
- 12 Cups lean beef steak strips (3 leans)
- 2 Cups Beef stock (1 condiment)
- 1 Cup Lettuce shredded (½ green)
- 10 Slices provolone cheese (1 healthy fat)
- 1 Onion, chopped

Directions:

1. In a slow cooker, add onion, beef, stock, pepper, and seasonings.
2. Cover, then cook at low heat for 6 or 8 hours.
3. Heat the tortillas for two minutes in the microwave.
4. Allow the air fryer to preheat to 350°F.
5. Remove the cheesesteak from the slow cooker, add 2-3 tablespoons of steak to the tortilla.
6. Add some cheese, roll the tortilla well, and place in a deep fryer basket.
7. Make all the tortillas you want.
8. Lightly brush with olive oil
9. Cook for 6-8 minutes.
10. Flip the tortillas over and brush more oil as needed.
11. Serve with chopped lettuce and enjoy.

Nutrition:

- Calories: 220
- Protein: 21g
- Fat: 16g

Chapter 8. Snacks and Party Food

87. Salmon Sandwich With Avocado and Egg

Preparation Time: 15 Minutes
Cooking Time: 10 Minutes
Servings: 4
Ingredients:

- 8 Ounces (250g) smoked salmon, thinly sliced
- 1 Medium (200g) ripe avocado, thinly sliced
- 4 Large poached eggs (about 60g each)
- 4 Slices whole wheat bread (about 30g each)
- 2 Cups (60g) arugula or baby rocket
- Salt and freshly ground black pepper

Directions:

1. Place one bread slice on a plate top with arugula, avocado, salmon, and poached egg—season with salt and pepper. Repeat the procedure for the remaining ingredients.
2. Serve and enjoy.

Nutrition:

- Calories: 310
- Fat: 18.2g
- Carbohydrates: 16.4g
- Protein: 21.3g
- Sodium: 383mg

88. Tasty Onion and Cauliflower Dip

Preparation Time: 20 Minutes
Cooking Time: 30 Minutes
Servings: 24
Ingredients:

- 1 and ½ Cups chicken stock
- 1 Cauliflower head, florets separated
- ¼ Cup mayonnaise
- ½ Cup yellow onion, chopped
- ¾ Cup cream cheese
- ½ Teaspoon chili powder
- ½ Teaspoon cumin, ground
- ½ Teaspoon garlic powder
- Salt and black pepper to the taste

Directions:

1. Put the stock in a pot, add cauliflower and onion, heat up over medium heat, and cook for 30 minutes.
2. Add chili powder, salt, pepper, cumin, and garlic powder and stir.
3. Also, add cream cheese and stir a bit until it melts.
4. Blend using an immersion blender and mix with the mayo.
5. Transfer to a bowl and keep in the fridge for 2 hours before you serve it.
6. Enjoy!

Nutrition:

- Calories: 40 kcal
- Protein: 1.23g
- Fat: 3.31g
- Carbohydrates: 1.66g
- Sodium: 72mg

89. Marinated Eggs

Preparation Time: 2 Hours and 10 Minutes
Cooking Time: 7 Minutes
Servings: 4
Ingredients:

- 6 Eggs
- 1 and ¼ Cups of water
- ¼ Cup unsweetened rice vinegar
- 2 Tablespoons coconut aminos
- Salt and black pepper to the taste
- 2 Garlic cloves, minced
- 1 Teaspoon stevia
- 4 Ounces cream cheese
- 1 Tablespoon chives, chopped

Directions:

1. Put the eggs in a pot, add water to cover, bring to a boil over medium heat, cover and cook for 7 minutes.
2. Rinse eggs with cold water and leave them aside to cool down.
3. In a bowl, mix one cup of water with coconut aminos, vinegar, stevia, and garlic and whisk well.
4. Put the eggs in this mix, cover with a kitchen towel, and leave them aside for 2 hours, rotating from time to time.
5. Peel eggs, cut in halves, and put egg yolks in a bowl.
6. Add ¼ cup water, cream cheese, salt, pepper, and chives, and stir well.
7. Stuff egg whites with this mix and serve them.
8. Enjoy!

Nutrition:

- Calories: 289 kcal
- Protein: 15.86g
- Fat: 22.62g
- Carbohydrates: 4.52g
- Sodium: 288mg

90. Pumpkin Muffins

Preparation Time: 10 Minutes
Cooking Time: 15 Minutes
Servings: 18
Ingredients:

- ¼ Cup sunflower seed butter
- ¾ Cup pumpkin puree
- 2 Tablespoons flaxseed meal
- ¼ Cup coconut flour
- ½ Cup erythritol
- ½ Teaspoon nutmeg, ground
- 1 Teaspoon cinnamon, ground
- ½ Teaspoon baking soda
- 1 Egg
- ½ Teaspoon baking powder
- A pinch of salt

Directions:

1. In a bowl, mix butter with pumpkin puree and egg and blend well.
2. Add flaxseed meal, coconut flour, erythritol, baking soda, baking powder, nutmeg, cinnamon, and a pinch of salt and stir well.
3. Spoon this into a greased muffin pan, introduce in the oven at 350 degrees Fahrenheit and bake for 15 minutes.
4. Leave muffins to cool down and serve them as a snack.
5. Enjoy!

Nutrition:

- Calories: 65 kcal
- Protein: 2.82g
- Fat: 5.42g
- Carbohydrates: 2.27g
- Sodium: 57mg

91. Salmon Spinach and Cottage Cheese Sandwich

Preparation Time: 15 Minutes
Cooking Time: 10 Minutes
Servings: 4
Ingredients:

- 4 Ounces (125g) cottage cheese
- 1/4 Cup (15g) chives, chopped
- 1 Teaspoon (5g) capers
- ½ Teaspoon (2.5g) grated lemon rind
- 4 (2 oz. or 60g) Smoked salmon
- 2 Cups (60g) loose baby spinach
- 1 Medium (110g) red onion, sliced thinly
- 8 Slices rye bread (about 30g each)
- Kosher salt and freshly ground black pepper

Directions:

1. Preheat your griddle or Panini press.
2. Mix together cottage cheese, chives, capers, and lemon rind in a small bowl.
3. Spread and divide the cheese mixture on four bread slices. Top with spinach, onion slices, and smoked salmon.
4. Cover with remaining bread slices.
5. Grill the sandwiches until golden and grill marks form on both sides.
6. Transfer to a serving dish.
7. Serve and enjoy.

Nutrition:

- Calories: 261
- Fat: 9.9g
- Carbohydrates: 22.9g
- Protein: 19.9g
- Sodium: 1226mg

92. Sausage and Cheese Dip

Preparation Time: 10 Minutes
Cooking Time: 130 Minutes
Servings: 28
Ingredients:

- 8 Ounces cream cheese
- A pinch of salt and black pepper
- 16 Ounces sour cream
- 8 Ounces pepper jack cheese, chopped
- 15 Ounces canned tomatoes mixed with habaneros
- 1-pound Italian sausage, ground
- ¼ Cup green onions, chopped

Directions:

1. Heat up a pan over medium heat, add sausage, stir and cook until it browns.
2. Add tomatoes, mix, stir and cook for 4 minutes more.
3. Add a pinch of salt, pepper, and green onions, stir and cook for 4 minutes.
4. Spread the pepper jack cheese on the bottom of your slow cooker.
5. Add cream cheese, sausage mix, and sour cream, cover, and cook on High for 2 hours.
6. Uncover your slow cooker, stir dip, transfer to a bowl, and serve.
7. Enjoy!

Nutrition:

- Calories: 132 kcal
- Protein: 6.79g
- Fat: 9.58g
- Carbohydrates: 6.22g
- Sodium: 362mg

93. Pesto Crackers

Preparation Time: 10 Minutes
Cooking Time: 17 Minutes
Servings: 6
Ingredients:

- ½ Teaspoon baking powder
- Salt and black pepper to the taste
- 1 and ¼ Cups almond flour
- ¼ Teaspoon basil dried one garlic clove, minced
- 2 Tablespoons basil pesto
- A pinch of cayenne pepper
- 3 Tablespoons ghee

Directions:

1. In a bowl, mix salt, pepper, baking powder, and almond flour.
2. Add garlic, cayenne, and basil and stir.
3. Add pesto and whisk.
4. Also, add ghee and mix your dough with your finger.
5. Spread this dough on a lined baking sheet, introduce in the oven at 325 degrees F and bake for 17 minutes.
6. Leave aside to cool down, cut your crackers, and serve them as a snack.
7. Enjoy!

Nutrition:

- Calories: 9 kcal
- Protein: 0.41g
- Fat: 0.14g
- Carbohydrates: 1.86g
- Sodium: 2mg

94. Bacon Cheeseburger

Preparation Time: 10 Minutes
Cooking Time: 30 Minutes
Servings: 4
Ingredients:

- 1 lb. Lean ground beef
- 1/4 Cup chopped yellow onion
- 1 Clove garlic, minced
- 1 Tbsp. yellow mustard
- 1 Tbsp. Worcestershire sauce
- ½ Tsp. salt
- Cooking spray
  4 Ultra-thin slices of cheddar cheese, cut into six equal-sized
- rectangular pieces
  3 Pieces of turkey bacon, each cut into eight evenly-sized
- rectangular pieces
- 24 Dill pickle chips
- 4-6 Green leaf
- Lettuce leaves, torn into 24 small square-shaped pieces
- 12 Cherry tomatoes, sliced in half

Directions:

1. Pre-heat oven to 400°F.
2. Combine the garlic, salt, onion, Worcestershire sauce, and beef in a medium-sized bowl, and mix well.
3. Form the mixture into 24 small meatballs.
4. Put meatballs onto a foil-lined baking sheet and cook for 12-15 minutes.
5. Leave the oven on.
6. Top every meatball with a piece of cheese, then go back to the oven until cheese melts for about 2 to 3 minutes.
7. Let the meatballs cool.
8. To assemble bites, on a toothpick, put a cheese-covered meatball, a piece of bacon, a piece of lettuce, pickle chip, and a tomato half.

Nutrition:

- Fat: 14g
- Cholesterol: 41mg
- Carbohydrates: 30g
- Protein: 15g

95. Cheeseburger Pie

Preparation Time: 20 Minutes
Cooking Time: 90 Minutes
Servings: 4
Ingredients:

- 1 Large spaghetti squash
- 1 lb. Lean ground beef
- 1/4 Cup diced onion
- 2 Eggs
- 1/3 Cup low-fat, plain Greek yogurt
- 2 Tablespoons tomato sauce
- ½ Tsp. Worcestershire sauce
- 2/3 Cups reduced-fat, shredded cheddar cheese
- 2 oz. Dill pickle slices
- Cooking spray

Directions:

1. Preheat oven to 400°F. Slice spaghetti squash in half lengthwise; dismiss pulp and seeds.
2. Spray insides with cooking spray.
3. Place squash halves cut-side-down onto a foil-lined baking sheet, and bake for 30 minutes.
4. Once cooked, let it cool before scraping squash flesh with a fork to remove spaghetti-like strands; set aside.
5. Push squash strands in the bottom and up sides of the greased pie pan, creating an even layer.
6. Meanwhile, set up pie filling.
7. In a lightly greased, medium-sized skillet, cook beef and onion over medium heat for 8 to 10 minutes, sometimes stirring, until meat is brown.
8. Drain and remove from heat.
9. In a medium-sized bowl, whisk together eggs, tomato sauce, Greek yogurt, and Worcestershire sauce. Stir in ground beef mixture.
10. Pour pie filling over the squash crust.
11. Sprinkle meat filling with cheese, and then top with dill pickle slices.
12. Bake for 40 minutes.

Nutrition:

- Calories: 409 Cal
- Fat: 24.49g
- Carbohydrates: 15.06g
- Protein: 30.69g

96. Smoked Salmon and Cheese on Rye Bread

Preparation Time: 15 Minutes
Cooking Time: 10 Minutes
Servings: 4
Ingredients:

- 8 Ounces (250g) smoked salmon, thinly sliced
- 1/3 Cup (85g) mayonnaise
- 2 Tablespoons (30ml) lemon juice
- 1 Tablespoon (15g) Dijon mustard
- 1 Teaspoon (3g) garlic, minced
- 4 Slices cheddar cheese (about 2 oz. or 30g each)
- 8 Slices rye bread (about 2 oz. or 30g each)
- 8 (15g) Romaine lettuce leaves
- Salt and freshly ground black pepper

Directions:

1. Mix together the mayonnaise, lemon juice, mustard, and garlic in a small bowl. Flavor with salt and pepper and set aside.
2. Spread dressing on four bread slices. Top with lettuce, salmon, and cheese. Cover with remaining rye bread slices.
3. Serve and enjoy.

Nutrition:

- Calories: 365
- Fat: 16.6g
- Carbohydrates: 31.6g
- Protein: 18.8g
- Sodium: 951mg

97. Chicken and Mushrooms

Preparation Time: 10 Minutes
Cooking Time: 15 Minutes
Servings: 6
Ingredients:

- 2 Chicken breasts
- 1 Cup of sliced white champignons
- 1 Cup of sliced green chilies
- ½ Cup scallions hacked
- 1 Teaspoon of chopped garlic
  1 Cup of low-fat cheddar shredded cheese (1-1,5 lb. grams fat
- / ounce)
- 1 Tablespoon of olive oil
- 1 Tablespoon of butter

Directions:

1. Fry the chicken breasts with olive oil.
2. When needed, add salt and pepper.
3. Grill the chicken breasts on a plate with a grill.
4. For every serving, weigh 4 ounces of chicken. (Make two servings, save leftovers for another meal).
5. In a buttered pan, stir in mushrooms, green peppers, scallions, and garlic until smooth and a little dark.
6. Place the chicken on a baking platter.
7. Cover with the mushroom combination.
8. Top on ham.
9. Place the cheese in a 350 oven until it melts.

Nutrition:

- Carbohydrates: 2g
- Protein: 23g
- Fat: 11g
- Cholesterol: 112mg
- Sodium: 198mg
- Potassium: 261mg

98. Chicken Enchilada Bake

Preparation Time: 20 Minutes
Cooking Time: 50 Minutes
Servings: 5
Ingredients:

- 5 oz. Shredded chicken breast (boil and shred ahead) or 99 percent fat-free white chicken can be used in a pan.
- 1 Can tomato paste
- 1 Low sodium chicken broth can be fat-free
- 1/4 Cup cheese with low-fat mozzarella
- 1 Tablespoon oil
- 1 Tbsp. of salt
  Ground cumin, chili powder, garlic powder, oregano, and
- onion powder (all to taste)
- 1 to 2 Zucchinis sliced longways (similar to lasagna noodles)
- into thin lines Sliced (optional) olives

Directions:

1. Add olive oil in a saucepan over medium/high heat, stir in tomato paste and seasonings, and heat in chicken broth for 2-3 min.
2. Stirring regularly to boil, turn heat to low for 15 min.
3. Set aside and cool to ambient temperature.
4. Dredge a zucchini strip through enchilada sauce and lay flat on the pan's bottom in a small baking pan.
5. Next, add the chicken a little less than 1/4 cup of enchilada sauce and mix it.
6. Attach the chicken to cover and end the baking tray.
7. Sprinkle some bacon over the chicken.

8. Add another layer of the soaked enchilada sauce zucchini (similar to lasagna making).
9. When needed, cover with the remaining cheese and olives on top—bake for 35 to 40 minutes.
10. Keep an eye on them.
11. When the cheese starts getting golden, cover with foil.
12. Serve and enjoy!

Nutrition:

- Calories: 312 Cal
- Carbohydrates: 21.3g
- Protein: 27g
- Fat: 10.2g

99. Salmon Feta and Pesto Wrap

Preparation Time: 15 Minutes
Cooking Time: 10 Minutes
Servings: 4
Ingredients:

- 8 Ounces (250g) smoked salmon fillet, thinly sliced
- 1 Cup (150g) feta cheese
- 8 (15g) Romaine lettuce leaves
- 4 (6-inch) Pita bread
- 1/4 Cup (60g) basil pesto sauce

Directions:

1. Place one pita bread on a plate. Top with lettuce, salmon, feta cheese, and pesto sauce. Fold or roll to enclose filling. Repeat the procedure for the remaining ingredients.
2. Serve and enjoy.

Nutrition:

- Calories: 379
- Fat: 17.7g
- Carbohydrates: 36.6g
- Protein: 18.4g
- Sodium: 554mg

100. Pan-Fried Trout

Preparation Time: 15 Minutes
Cooking Time: 10 Minutes
Servings: 4
Ingredients:

- 1 ¼ Pounds trout fillets
- 1/3 Cup white, or yellow, cornmeal
- ¼ Teaspoon anise seeds
- ¼ Teaspoon black pepper
- ½ Cup minced cilantro, or parsley
- Vegetable cooking spray
- Lemon wedges

Directions:

1. Coat the fish with combined cornmeal, spices, and cilantro, pressing them gently into the fish. Spray a large skillet with cooking spray; heat over medium heat until hot.
2. Add fish and cook until it is tender and flakes with a fork, about 5 minutes on each side. Serve with lemon wedges.

Nutrition:

- Calories: 207
- Total Carbohydrates: 19g
- Cholesterol: 27mg
- Total Fat: 16g
- Fiber: 4g
- Protein: 18g

101. Glazed Bananas in Phyllo Nut Cups

Preparation Time: 30 Minutes
Cooking Time: 45 Minutes
Servings: 6 Servings
Ingredients:

- 3/4 Cups shelled pistachios
- ½ Cup sugar
- 1 Teaspoon. ground cinnamon
- 4 Sheets phyllo dough (14 inches x 9 inches)
- 1/4 Cup butter, melted

Sauce:

- 3/4 Cup butter, cubed
- 3/4 Cup packed brown sugar
- 3 Medium-firm bananas, sliced
- 1/4 Teaspoon. ground cinnamon
- 3 to 4 Cups vanilla ice cream

Directions:

1. Finely chop sugar and pistachios in a food processor; move to a bowl, then mix in cinnamon. Slice each phyllo sheet into six four-inch squares, get rid of the trimmings. Pile the squares, then use plastic wrap to cover.
2. Slather melted butter on each square one at a time, then scatter a heaping tablespoonful of pistachio mixture. Pile three squares, flip each at an angle to misalign the corners. Force each stack on the sides and bottom of an oiled eight ounces custard cup. Bake for 15-20 minutes in a 350 degrees F oven until golden; cool for 5 minutes. Move to a wire rack to cool completely.
3. Melt and boil brown sugar and butter in a saucepan to make the sauce; lower heat. Mix in cinnamon and bananas gently; heat completely. Put ice cream in the phyllo cups until full, then put banana sauce on top. Serve right away.

Nutrition:

- Calories: 735
- Total Carbohydrate: 82g
- Cholesterol: 111mg
- Total Fat: 45g
- Fiber: 3g
- Protein: 7g
- Sodium: 468mg

102. Salmon Cream Cheese and Onion on Bagel

Preparation Time: 15 Minutes
Cooking Time: 10 Minutes
Servings: 4
Ingredients:

- 8 Ounces (250g) smoked salmon fillet, thinly sliced
- ½ Cup (125g) cream cheese
- 1 Medium (110g) onion, thinly sliced
- 4 Bagels (about 80g each), split
- 2 Tablespoons (7g) fresh parsley, chopped
- Freshly ground black pepper, to taste

Directions:

4. Spread the cream cheese on each bottom's half of bagels. Top with salmon and onion, season with pepper, sprinkle with parsley and then cover with bagel tops.
5. Serve and enjoy.

Nutrition:

- Calories: 309
- Fat: 14.1g
- Carbohydrates: 32.0g
- Protein: 14.7g
- Sodium: 571mg

219. Salmon Apple Salad Sandwich

Preparation Time: 15 Minutes
Cooking Time: 10 Minutes
Servings: 4
Ingredients:

- 4 Ounces (125g) canned pink salmon, drained and flaked
- 1 Medium (180g) red apple, cored and diced
- 1 Celery stalk (about 60g), chopped
- 1 Shallot (about 40g), finely chopped
- 1/3 Cup (85g) light mayonnaise
- 8 Whole grain bread slices (about 30g each), toasted
- 8 (15g) Romaine lettuce leaves
- Salt and freshly ground black pepper

Directions:

1. Combine the salmon, apple, celery, shallot, and mayonnaise in a mixing bowl—season with salt and pepper.
2. Place one bread slice on a plate, top with lettuce and salmon salad, and then cover it with another slice of bread—repeat the procedure for the remaining ingredients.
3. Serve and enjoy.

Nutrition:

- Calories: 315
- Fat: 11.3g
- Carbohydrates: 40.4g
- Protein: 15.1g
- Sodium: 469mg

103. Greek Baklava

Preparation Time: 20 Minutes
Cooking Time: 20 Minutes
Servings: 18
Ingredients:

- 1 (16 oz.) Package phyllo dough
- 1 lb. Chopped nuts
- 1 Cup butter
- 1 Teaspoon ground cinnamon
- 1 Cup water
- 1 Cup white sugar
- 1 Teaspoon vanilla extract
- ½ Cup honey

Directions:

1. Preheat the oven to 175°C or 350°Fahrenheit. Spread butter on the sides and bottom of a 9- by 13-inch pan.
2. Chop the nuts, then mix with cinnamon; set it aside. Unfurl the phyllo dough, then halve the whole stack to fit the pan. Use a damp cloth to cover the phyllo to prevent drying as you proceed. Put two phyllo sheets in the pan, then butter well. Repeat to make eight layered phyllo sheets. Scatter 2-3 tablespoons of the nut mixture over the sheets, then place two more phyllo sheets on top, butter, sprinkle with nuts—layer as you go. The final layer should be six to eight phyllo sheets deep.
3. Make square or diamond shapes with a sharp knife up to the bottom of the pan. You can slice into four long rows for diagonal shapes. Bake until crisp and golden for 50 minutes.
4. Meanwhile, boil water and sugar until the sugar melts to make the sauce; mix in honey and vanilla. Let it simmer for 20 minutes.
5. Take the baklava out of the oven, then drizzle with sauce right away; cool. Serve the baklava in cupcake papers. You can also freeze them without cover. The baklava will turn soggy when wrapped.

Nutrition:

- Calories: 393
- Total Carbohydrate: 37.5g
- Cholesterol: 27mg
- Total Fat: 25.9g
- Protein: 6.1g
- Sodium: 196mg

104. Easy Salmon Burger

Preparation Time: 15 minutes
Cooking Time: 15 minutes
Servings: 6
Ingredients:

- 16 Ounces (450g) pink salmon, minced
- 1 Cup (250g) prepared mashed potatoes
- 1 Medium (110g) onion, chopped
- 1 Stalk celery (about 60g), finely chopped
- 1 Large egg (about 60g), lightly beaten
- 2 Tablespoons (7g) fresh cilantro, chopped
- 1 Cup (100g) breadcrumbs
- Vegetable oil, for deep frying
- Salt and freshly ground black pepper

Directions:

1. Combine the salmon, mashed potatoes, onion, celery, egg, and cilantro in a mixing bowl. Season to taste and mix thoroughly. Spoon about 2 Tablespoons of the mixture, roll in breadcrumbs, and then form into small patties.
2. Heat oil in a non-stick frying pan. Cook your salmon patties for 5 minutes on each side or until golden brown and crispy.
3. Serve in burger buns and with coleslaw on the side if desired.
4. Enjoy.

Nutrition:

- Calories: 230
- Fat: 7.9g
- Carbs: 20.9g
- Protein: 18.9g
- Sodium: 298mg

105. White Bean Dip

Preparation Time: 10 Minutes
Cooking Time: 0 Minutes
Servings: 4
Ingredients:

- 15 Ounces canned white beans, drained and rinsed
- 6 Ounces canned artichoke hearts, drained and quartered
- 4 Garlic cloves, minced
- 1 Tablespoon basil, chopped
- 2 Tablespoons olive oil
- Juice of ½ lemon
- Zest of ½ lemon, grated
- Salt and black pepper to the taste

Directions:

1. In your food processor, combine the beans with the artichokes and the rest of the ingredients except the oil and pulse well.
2. Add the oil gradually, pulse the mix again, divide into cups and serve as a party dip.

Nutrition:

- Calories: 274
- Fat: 11.7g
- Fiber: 6.5g
- Carbs: 18.5g
- Protein: 16.5g

106. Grilled Salmon Burger

Preparation Time: 15 Minutes
Cooking Time: 10 Minutes
Servings: 4
Ingredients:

- 16 Ounces (450g) pink salmon fillet, minced
- 1 Cup (250g) prepared mashed potatoes
- 1 Shallot (about 40g), chopped
- 1 Large egg (about 60g), lightly beaten
- 2 Tablespoons (7g) fresh coriander, chopped
- 4 Hamburger buns (about 60g each), split
- 1 Large tomato (about 150g), sliced
- 8 (15g) Romaine lettuce leaves
- 1/4 Cup (60g) mayonnaise
- Salt and freshly ground black pepper
- Cooking oil spray

Directions:

1. Combine the salmon, mashed potatoes, shallot, egg, and coriander in a mixing bowl—season with salt and pepper.
2. Spoon about two tablespoons of mixture and form into patties.
3. Preheat your grill or griddle on high—grease with cooking oil spray.
4. Grill the salmon patties for 4-5 minutes on each side or until cooked through. Transfer to a clean plate and cover to keep warm.
5. Spread some mayonnaise on the bottom half of the buns. Top with lettuce, salmon patty, and tomato. Cover with bun tops.
6. Serve and enjoy.

Nutrition:

- Calories: 395
- Fat: 18.0g
- Carbohydrates: 38.8g
- Protein: 21.8g
- Sodium: 383mg

Chapter 9. Desserts Recipes

107. Chocolate Bars

Preparation Time: 10 Minutes
Cooking Time: 20 Minutes
Servings: 16
Ingredients:

- 15 oz. Cream cheese softened
- 15 oz. Unsweetened dark chocolate
- 1 Tsp. Vanilla
- 10 Drops liquid stevia

Directions:

1. Grease an 8-inch square dish and set it aside.
2. In a saucepan, dissolve chocolate over low heat.
3. Add stevia and vanilla and stir well.
4. Remove the pan from heat and set it aside.
5. Add cream cheese into the blender and blend until smooth.
6. Add the melted chocolate mixture into the cream cheese and blend until just combined.
7. Transfer mixture into the prepared dish and spread evenly, and place in the refrigerator until firm.
8. Slice and serve.

Nutrition:

- Calories: 230
- Fat: 24g
- Carbs: 7.5g
- Sugar: 0.1g
- Protein: 6g
- Cholesterol: 29mg

108. Blueberry Muffins

Preparation Time: 15 Minutes
Cooking Time: 35 Minutes
Servings: 12
Ingredients:

- 2 Eggs
- ½ Cup fresh blueberries
- 1 Cup heavy cream
- 2 Cups almond flour
- 1/4 Tsp. lemon zest
- ½ Tsp. lemon extract
- 1 Tsp. baking powder
- 5 Drops stevia
- 1/4 Cup butter, melted

Directions:

1. Heat the cooker to 350°F. Line muffin tin with cupcake liners and set aside.
2. Add eggs into the bowl and whisk until mix.
3. Add remaining ingredients and mix to combine.
4. Pour mixture into the prepared muffin tin and bake for 25 minutes.
5. Serve and enjoy.

Nutrition:

- Calories: 190
- Fat: 17g
- Carbs: 5g
- Sugar: 1g
- Protein: 5g
- Cholesterol: 55mg

109. Chocolate Fondue

Preparation Time: 5 Minutes
Cooking Time: 10 Minutes
Servings: 2
Ingredients:

- 1 Cup water
- ½ Tsp. sugar
- ½ Cup coconut cream
- ¾ Cup dark chocolate, chopped

Directions:

1. Pour the water into your Instant Pot.
2. To a heatproof bowl, add the chocolate, sugar, and coconut cream.
3. Place in the Instant Pot.
4. Seal the lid, select MANUAL, and cook for 2 minutes. When ready, do a quick release and carefully open the lid. Stir well and serve immediately.

Nutrition:

- Calories: 216
- Fat: 17g
- Carbs: 11g
- Protein: 2g

110. Apple Crisp

Preparation Time: 10 Minutes
Cooking Time: 13 Minutes
Servings: 2
Ingredients:

- 2 Apples, sliced into chunks
- 1 Tsp. Cinnamon
- ¼ Cup rolled oats
- 1/4 Cup brown sugar
- ½ Cup of water

Directions:

1. Put all the listed ingredients in the pot and mix well.
2. Seal the pot, choose MANUAL mode, and cook at HIGH pressure for 8 minutes.
3. Release the pressure naturally and let sit for 5 minutes or until the sauce has thickened.
4. Serve and enjoy.

Nutrition:

- Calories: 218
- Fat: 5mg
- Carbs: 54g

111. Yogurt Mint

Preparation Time: 5 Minutes
Cooking Time: 10 Minutes
Servings: 2
Ingredients:

- 1 Cup of water
- 5 Cups of milk
- ¾ Cup plain yogurt
- ¼ Cup fresh mint
- 1 Tbsp. maple syrup

Directions:

1. Add one water cup to the Instant Pot Pressure Cooker.
2. Press the STEAM function button and adjust it to 1 minute.
3. Once done, add the milk, then press the YOGURT function button and allow boiling.
4. Add yogurt and fresh mint, then stir well.
5. Pour into a glass and add maple syrup.
6. Enjoy.

Nutrition:

- Calories: 25
- Fat: 0.5g
- Carbs: 5g
- Protein: 2g

112. Raspberry Compote

Preparation Time: 11 Minutes
Cooking Time: 30 Minutes
Servings: 2
Ingredients:

- 1 Cup raspberries
- ½ Cup Swerve
- 1 Tsp. freshly grated lemon zest
- 1 Tsp. vanilla extract
- 2 Cups water

Directions:

1. Press the SAUTÉ button on your Instant Pot, then add all the listed ingredients.
2. Stir well and pour in one cup of water.
3. Cook for 5 minutes, continually stirring, then pour in 1 more cup of water and press the CANCEL button.
4. Secure the lid properly, press the MANUAL button, and set the timer to 15 minutes on LOW pressure.
5. When the timer buzzes, press the CANCEL button and release the pressure naturally for 10minutes.
6. Move the pressure handle to the "venting" position to release any remaining pressure and open the lid.
7. Let it cool before serving.

Nutrition:

- Calories: 48
- Fat: 0.5g
- Carbs: 5g
- Protein: 1g

113. Braised Apples

Preparation Time: 5 Minutes
Cooking Time: 12 Minutes
Servings: 2
Ingredients:

- 2 Cored apples
- ½ Cup of water
- ½ Cup red wine
- 3 Tbsp. sugar
- ½ Tsp. ground cinnamon

Directions:

1. In the bottom of the Instant Pot, add the water and place the apples.
2. Pour wine on top and sprinkle with sugar and cinnamon. Close the lid carefully and cook for 10 minutes at HIGH PRESSURE.
3. When done, do a quick pressure release.
4. Transfer the apples onto serving plates and top with cooking liquid.
5. Serve immediately.

Nutrition:

- Calories: 245
- Fat: 0.5g
- Carbs: 53g
- Protein: 1g

114. Rice Pudding

Preparation Time: 5 Minutes
Cooking Time: 12 Minutes
Servings: 2
Ingredients:

- ½ Cup short grain rice
- ¼ Cup of sugar
- 1 Cinnamon stick
- 1½ Cup milk
- 1 Slice lemon peel
- Salt to taste

Directions:

1. Rinse the rice under cold water.
2. Put the rice, milk, cinnamon stick, sugar, salt, and lemon peel inside the Instant Pot Pressure Cooker.
3. Close the lid, lock it in place, and make sure to seal the valve. Press the PRESSURE button and cook for 10 minutes on HIGH.
4. When the timer beeps, choose the QUICK PRESSURE release. This will take about 2 minutes.
5. Remove the lid. Open the pressure cooker and discard the lemon peel and cinnamon stick. Spoon in a serving bowl and serve.

Nutrition:

- Calories: 111
- Fat: 6g
- Carbs: 21g
- Protein: 3g

115. Rhubarb Dessert

Preparation Time: 4 Minutes
Cooking Time: 5 Minutes
Servings: 2
Ingredients:

- 3 Cups rhubarb, chopped
- 1 Tbsp. ghee, melted
- 1/3 Cup water
- 1 Tbsp. stevia
- 1 Tsp. vanilla extract

Directions:

1. Put all the listed ingredients in your Instant Pot, cover, and cook on HIGH for 5 minutes.
2. Divide into small bowls and serve cold.
3. Enjoy!

Nutrition:

- Calories: 83
- Fat: 2g
- Carbs: 2g
- Protein: 2g

116. Wine Figs

Preparation Time: 5 Minutes
Cooking Time: 3 Minutes
Servings: 2
Ingredients:

- ½ Cup pine nuts
- 1 Cup red wine
- 1 lb. Figs
- Sugar, as needed

Directions:

1. Slowly pour the wine and sugar into the Instant Pot.
2. Arrange the trivet inside it; place the figs over it. Close the lid and lock. Ensure that you have sealed the valve to avoid leakage.
3. Press MANUAL mode and set the timer to 3 minutes.
4. After the timer reads zero, you have to press CANCEL and quick-release pressure.
5. Carefully remove the lid.
6. Divide figs into bowls, and drizzle wine from the pot over them.
7. Top with pine nuts and enjoy.

Nutrition:

- Calories: 95
- Fat: 3g
- Carbs: 5g
- Protein: 2g

117. Chia Pudding

Preparation Time: 20 Minutes
Cooking Time: 0 Minutes
Servings: 2
Ingredients:

- 4 Tbsp. chia seeds
- 1 Cup unsweetened coconut milk
- ½ Cup raspberries

Directions:

1. Add raspberry and coconut milk into a blender and blend until smooth.
2. Pour mixture into a glass jar.
3. Add chia seeds in a jar and stir well.
4. Seal the jar with a lid and shake well and place in the refrigerator for 3 hours.
5. Serve chilled and enjoy.

Nutrition:

- Calories: 360
- Fat: 33g
- Carbs: 13g
- Sugar: 5g
- Protein: 6g
  Cholesterol: 0mg

Chapter 10. Air Fryer Meals and Breakfast Recipes

118. Cloud Focaccia Bread Breakfast

Difficulty: Difficult
Preparation Time: 10 Minutes
Cooking Time: 30 Minutes
Servings: 2
Ingredients:

- 2 Medium eggs, separate yolk, and white (1 healthy fat)
- 1½ Tbsp. Cream cheese, low fat (1 healthy fat)
- ½ Package sweetener, no-calorie (½ condiment)
- ¼ Tsp. Tartar cream (1/4 condiment)

For Focaccia Bread:

- ½ Tsp. Olive oil
- ½ Tsp. Rosemary (½ green)
- 1/8 Tsp. Salt (1/4 condiment)

Directions:

1. Combine thoroughly cream cheese, egg yolks, and the sweetener in a medium bowl.
2. Beat the egg whites in a large bowl along with tartar cream until the whites become stiff peaks.
3. Now carefully fold the yolk mixture into the egg whites without breaking the whites.
4. Line a parchment paper in the air fryer baking tray and place four scoops of the mixture without overlapping one another.
5. Set the temperature to 150°C and bake for 20 minutes.
6. Take out the bread, brush olive oil on top and sprinkle Rosemary and salt.
7. Place it again into the air fryer and bake for further 10 minutes until the top becomes golden brown.
8. After baking, allow it to cool down before serving.

Nutrition:

- Calories: 90
- Fat: 6.5g
- Protein: 6g

119. Cloud Garlic Bread Breakfast

Difficulty: Difficult
Preparation Time: 10 Minutes
Cooking Time: 30 Minutes
Servings: 2
Ingredients:

- 2 Eggs, medium (separate yolk and white) (1 healthy fat)
- 1½ Tbsp. Cream cheese, low fat (1 healthy fat)
- ½ Packet Sweetener, no-calorie (½ condiment)
- ¼ Tsp. Tartar cream (1/4 condiment)

For Garlic Bread:

- 1 Tsp. Butter, unsalted, melted (½ healthy fat)
- 1/8 Tsp. Garlic powder (1/4 condiment)
- ¼ Tsp. Italian seasoning (1/4 condiment)
- 1/8 Tsp. Salt (1/4 condiment)

Directions:

1. Combine thoroughly cream cheese, egg yolks, and the sweetener in a medium bowl.
2. Beat the egg whites in a large bowl along with tartar cream until the whites become stiff peaks.
3. Now carefully fold the yolk mixture into the egg whites without breaking the whites.
4. Line a parchment paper in the air fryer baking tray and place four scoops of the mixture without overlapping one another.
5. Set the temperature to 150°C and bake for 20 minutes.
6. Take out the bread, and brush butter on top and sprinkle the seasoning, garlic powder, and salt.
7. Place it again into the air fryer and bake for further 10 minutes until the top becomes golden brown.
8. After baking, allow it to cool before serving.

Nutrition:

- Calories: 115
- Fat: 8.8g
- Protein: 6g

120. Cheesy Broccoli Bites

Difficulty: Average
Preparation Time: 5 Minutes
Cooking Time: 40 Minutes
Servings: 2
Ingredients:

- 3 Cups Frozen broccoli (2greens)
- ¼ Cup Scallions, thinly sliced (½ green)
- 2 Eggs (1 healthy fat)
- 1 Cup Cottage cheese (½ healthy fat)
- ¾ Cup Mozzarella cheese, grated (½ healthy fat)
- ¼ Cup Parmesan cheese, shredded (1/4 healthy fat)
- 1 Tsp. Olive oil (½ condiment)
- ½ Tsp. Garlic powder (½ condiment)
- 1/8 Tsp. Salt (1/4 condiment)
- 2 Cups Water (1 healthy fat)

Directions:

1. Preheat the air fryer to 190°C.
2. Place the broccoli in an air fryer, save bowl, and pour water.
3. Air fryer it for 10 minutes until the broccoli becomes tender.
4. Drain the water and transfer the broccoli into the blender.
5. Blitz it until it chopped well.
6. Now add cottage cheese, scallions, parmesan, mozzarella, eggs, olive oil, salt, and garlic into the blender.
7. Pulse it until it gets mixed well.
8. Transfer it to 12 muffin tins evenly after greasing them.
9. Place it in the air fryer and bake for 30 minutes until the filling becomes firm and its top turns to a golden brown.
10. After baking, remove them from the air fryer.
11. Allow it to settle down the heat and serve.

Nutrition:

- Calories: 366
- Fat: 15.1g
- Protein: 41g

121. Portabella Mushrooms Stuffed With Cheese

Difficulty: Difficult
Preparation Time: 15 Minutes
Cooking Time: 17 Minutes
Servings: 2
Ingredients:

- 4 Portabella mushroom caps, large (2 leans)
- 1 Tbsp. Soy sauce (½ condiment)
- 1 Tbsp. Lemon juice (½ condiment)
- 1 Tsp. Olive oil, divided (1/4 condiment)
- 2 Cups Mozzarella cheese, low fat, grated (1 healthy fat)
- ½ Cup Tomato, fresh, diced (½ green)
- 1 Garlic Clove, finely grated (1/4green)
- 1 Tbsp. Cilantro, fresh, chopped (1/4green)

Directions:

1. Make bowls by scooping the flesh from the interior of the mushroom caps.
2. Set the air fryer temperature to 200°C and preheat.
3. Mix the soy sauce, lemon juice, and half a portion of olive oil in a small bowl.
4. Marinate the mixture on the mushroom cap both inside and outside.
5. Line foil-coated baking paper in the air fryer tray.
6. Place the marinated mushroom cap in the tray and bake for 10 minutes until they become tender.
7. Now combine tomatoes, mozzarella, garlic, remaining olive oil, and Italian seasoning in a medium bowl.
8. Fill the mushroom caps with the mixture evenly.
9. Bake it in the air fryer for 7 minutes until the cheese starts to melt.
10. Sprinkle cilantro on top and serve.

Nutrition:

- Calories: 250
- Fat: 4.4g
- Protein: 40g

122. Bell-Pepper Wrapped in Tortilla

Difficulty: Easy
Preparation Time: 5 Minutes
Cooking Time: 15 Minutes
Servings: 1
Ingredients:

- 1/4 Small red bell pepper (½ greens)
- 1/4 Tablespoon water (½ condiment)
- 1 Large tortilla (1 healthy fat)
- 1-piece Commercial vegan nuggets, chopped (3 leans)
- Mixed greens for garnish (6greens)

Directions:

1. Preheat the Instant Crisp Air Fryer to 400°F.
2. In a skillet heated over medium heat, water sautés the vegan nuggets and bell pepper. Set aside.
3. Place filling inside the corn tortilla.
4. Fold the tortilla, place them inside the Instant Crisp Air Fryer, and cook for 15 minutes until the tortilla wrap is crispy.
5. Serve with mixed greens on top.

Nutrition:

- Calories: 548
- Fat: 21g
- Protein: 46g

123. Air Fried Cauliflower Ranch Chips

Difficulty: Easy
Preparation Time: 5 Minutes
Cooking Time: 12 Minutes
Servings: 2
Ingredients:

- ½ Cup Raw cauliflower, grated (1/4green)
- ¼ Tsp. Parsley (1/8green)
- ¼ Tsp. Basil (1/8green)
- ¼ Tsp. Dill (1/8green)
- ¼ Tsp. Chives (1/8green)
- ¼ Tsp. Garlic powder (1/8 condiment)
- ¼ Tsp. Onion powder (1/8 condiment)
- ¼ Tsp. Pepper, ground (1/8 condiment)
- ¼ Cup Parmesan cheese (1/8 healthy fat)
- Cooking spray as required (½ healthy fat)

Directions:

1. Preheat the air fryer to 230°C.

2. Using a medium bowl, mix all the ingredients.
3. Line the air fryer baking tray with parchment paper.
4. Scoop one tablespoon of mixture and place it on the parchment paper without overlapping one another.
5. Bake for 12 minutes by flipping side halfway through.
6. Serve hot.

Nutrition:

- Calories: 65
- Fat: 3.6g
- Protein: 4g

124. Brine & Spinach Egg Air Fried Muffins

Difficulty: Difficult
Preparation Time: 10 Minutes
Cooking Time: 25 Minutes
Servings: 2
Ingredients:
For the Egg Muffin:

- 4 Eggs (2 healthy fat)
- 1 Cup Liquid egg whites (½ healthy fat)
- ¼ Cup Greek yogurt, plain, low fat (½ healthy fat)
- ¼ Tsp. Salt (1/4 condiment)

For Brie, Spinach & Mushroom Mix:

- 1 oz. Brie (½ green)
- 5 oz. Spinach, frozen, coarsely chopped (2greens)
- 1 Cup Mushrooms, chopped (½ green)

Directions:

1. Thaw the frozen spinach for 10 minutes.
2. Wash all the vegetables separately and pat dry.
3. Preheat the air fryer to 190°C.
4. In a large bowl, combine Greek yogurt, egg whites, eggs, cheese, and salt.
5. Add all the vegetables to the bowl, mix, and combine well.
6. Take 12 muffin tins and lightly spray with cooking oil.
7. Transfer the mixture evenly into the muffin tins.
8. Place them in the air fryer and bake for 25 minutes until the center portion becomes hard.
9. Do a toothpick test by inserting it in the center and check if it comes out clean.
10. Take it out from the air fryer and allow it to settle down the heat before serving.
11. Enjoy your muffin.

Nutrition:

- Calories: 278
- Fat: 13.1g
- Protein: 33g

125. Coconut Battered Cauliflower Bites

Difficulty: Average
Preparation Time: 5 Minutes
Cooking Time: 20 Minutes
Servings: 1
Ingredients:

- Salt and pepper to taste (2 condiments)
  1 Flax egg or one tablespoon flaxseed meal + 3 tablespoon
- water (1 healthy fat)
- 1 Small cauliflower, cut into florets (2greens)
- 1 Teaspoon mixed spice (1 condiment)
- ½ Teaspoon mustard powder (1 condiment)
- 2 Tablespoons maple syrup (2 healthy fats)
- 1 Clove of garlic, minced (1green)
- 2 Tablespoons soy sauce (2 condiments)
- 1/3 Cup oats flour (½ healthy fat)
- 1/3 Cup plain flour (½ healthy fat)
- 1/3 Cup desiccated coconut (½ lean)

Directions:

1. In a mixing bowl, mix oats, flour, and desiccated coconut. Season with salt and pepper to taste. Set aside.
2. In another bowl, place the flax egg and add a pinch of salt to taste. Set aside.
3. Season the cauliflower with mixed spice and mustard powder.
4. Dredge the florets in the flax egg first, then in the flour mixture.
5. Place inside the Instant Crisp Air Fryer, lock the air fryer lid, and cook at 400°F or 15 minutes.
6. Meanwhile, place the maple syrup, garlic, and soy sauce in a saucepan and heat over medium flame. Wait for it to boil and adjust the heat to low until the sauce thickens.
7. After 15 minutes, take out the Instant Crisp Air Fryer's florets and place them in the saucepan.
8. Toss to coat the florets and place inside the Instant Crisp Air Fryer and cook for another 5 minutes.

Nutrition:

- Calories: 154
- Fat: 2.3g
- Protein: 4.6g

126. Crispy Roasted Broccoli

Difficulty: Easy
Preparation Time: 10 minutes
Cooking Time: 8 minutes
Servings: 1
Ingredients:

- 1/4 Tsp. Masala (½ condiment)
- ½ Tsp. Red chili powder (1 condiment)
- ½ Tsp. Salt (1 condiment)
- 1/4 Tsp. Turmeric powder (½ condiment)
- 1 Tbsp. Chickpea flour (1 healthy fat)
- 1 Tbsp. Yogurt (2 healthy fats)
- ½ Pound broccoli (1green)

Directions:

1. Cut broccoli up into florets. Immerse in a bowl of water with two teaspoons of salt for at least half an hour to remove impurities.
2. Take out broccoli florets from water and let drain. Wipe down thoroughly.
3. Mix all other ingredients to create a marinade.
4. Toss broccoli florets in the marinade. Cover and chill for 15-30 minutes.
5. Preheat the Instant Crisp Air Fryer to 390 degrees. Place marinated broccoli florets into the fryer, lock the air fryer lid, set the temperature to 350°F, and set the time to 10 minutes. Florets will be crispy when done.

Nutrition:

- Calories: 96
- Fat: 1.3g
- Protein: 7g

127. Crispy Cauliflowers

Difficulty: Easy
Preparation Time: 10 Minutes
Cooking Time: 10 Minutes
Servings: 4
Ingredients:

- 2 Cup cauliflower florets, diced (6greens)
- ½ Cup almond flour (1 healthy fat)
- ½ Cup coconut flour (1 healthy fat)
- Salt and pepper to taste (½ condiment)
- 1 Tsp. Mixed herbs (1green)
- 1 Tsp. Chives, chopped (1green)
- 1 Egg (1 lean)
- 1 Tsp. Cumin (1 condiment)
- ½ Tsp. Garlic powder (1 condiment)
- 1 Cup water (1 condiment)
- Oil for frying (1 condiment)

Directions:

1. Combine the egg, salt, garlic, water, cumin, chives, mixed herbs, pepper, and flour in a mixing bowl.
2. Stir in the cauliflower to the mixture and then fry them in oil until they become golden in color.
3. Serve.

Nutrition:

- Protein: 3.3g
- Fat: 10.4g
- Calories: 259

128. Red Pepper & Kale Air Fried Egg Muffins

Difficulty: Average
Preparation Time: 10 Minutes
Cooking Time: 25 Minutes
Servings: 2
Ingredients:
For the Egg Muffin:

- 4 Eggs (1 healthy fat)
- 1 Cup Liquid egg whites (½ healthy fat)
- ¼ Cup Greek yogurt, plain, low fat (1/4 healthy fat)
- ¼ Tsp. Salt (1/4 condiment)

For the Red Bell Pepper, Goat Cheese & Kale Mix:

- 6 oz. Red bell pepper, cored and chopped (3greens)
- 5 oz. Kale, frozen, chopped (2greens)
- 1 oz. Goat cheese (½ healthy fat)

Directions:

1. Thaw the frozen cauliflower rice for 10 minutes.
2. Preheat the air fryer to 190°C.
3. In a large bowl, combine Greek yogurt, egg whites, eggs, cheese, and salt.
4. Add all the vegetables to the bowl mix to combine well.
5. Take 12 muffin tins and lightly spray with cooking oil.
6. Transfer the mixture evenly into the muffin tins.
7. Place them in the air fryer and bake for 25 minutes until the center portion becomes hard.
8. Do a toothpick test by inserting it in the center and check if it comes out clean.
9. Take it out from the air fryer and allow it to settle down the heat before serving.
10. Enjoy your muffin.

Nutrition:

- Calories: 323
- Fat: 15.4g
- Protein: 34g

Chapter 11. Side Dish Recipes

129. Low Carb Air-Fried Calzones

Preparation Time: 15 Minutes
Cooking Time: 27 Minutes
Servings: 2
Ingredients:

- 1/3 Cup cooked chicken breast (shredded)
- One teaspoon olive oil
- 3 Cups Spinach leaves (baby)
- Whole-wheat pizza dough, freshly prepared
- 1/3 Cup Marinara sauce (lower-sodium)
- 1/4 Cup Diced red onion
- 6 Tbsp. Skim mozzarella cheese
- Cooking spray

Directions:

1. In a medium skillet, over a medium flame, add oil, onions. Sauté until soft. Then add spinach leaves, cook until wilted. Turn off the heat and add chicken and marinara sauce.
2. Cut the dough into two pieces.
3. Add 1/4 of the spinach mix on each circle dough piece.
4. Add skim shredded cheese on top. Fold the dough over and crimp the edges.
5. Spray the calzones with cooking spray.
6. Put calzones in the air fryer. Cook for 12 minutes, at 325°F, until the dough is light brown. Turn the calzone over and cook for eight more minutes.

Nutrition:

- Calories: 348
- Fat: 12g
- Protein: 21g
- Carbohydrate: 18g

130. Air-Fried Tortilla Hawaiian Pizza

Preparation Time: 10 Minutes
Cooking Time: 20 Minutes
Servings: 1
Ingredients:

- Mozzarella Cheese
- Tortilla wrap
- 1 Tbsp. Tomato sauce

Toppings:

- 2 Tbsp. Cooked chicken shredded or hotdog
- 3 Tbsp. Pineapple pieces
- Half slice of ham, cut into pieces
- Cheese slice cut into pieces

Directions:

1. Lay a tortilla flat on a plate, add tomato sauce, and spread it.
2. Add some shredded mozzarella, add toppings. Top with cheese slices
3. Put in the air fryer and cook for five or ten minutes at 160 C.
4. Take out from the air fryer and slice it. Serve hot with baby spinach.

Nutrition:

- Calories: 178
- Proteins: 21g
- Carbs: 15g
- Fat: 15g

131. Tasty Kale & Celery Crackers

Preparation Time: 10 Minutes
Cooking Time: 20 Minutes
Servings: 2
Ingredients:

- 1 Cup of flax seeds, ground
- 1 Cup flax seeds, soaked overnight and drained
- 2 Bunches kale, chopped
- 1 Bunch basil, chopped
- ½ Bunch celery, chopped
- 2 Garlic cloves, minced
- 1/3 Cup olive oil

Directions:

1. Mix the ground flaxseed with celery, kale, basil, and garlic in your food processor and mix well.
2. Add the oil and soaked flaxseed, then mix again, scatter in the pan of your air fryer, break into medium crackers and cook for 20 minutes at 380 degrees F.
3. Serve as an appetizer and break into cups.
4. Enjoy

Nutrition:

- Calories: 143
- Fat: 1g
- Fiber: 2g
- Carbs: 8g
- Protein: 4g

132. Air Fryer Personal Mini Pizza

Preparation Time: 2 Minutes
Cooking Time: 5 Minutes
Servings: 1
Ingredients:

- 1/4 Cup Sliced olives
- 1 Pita bread
- 1 Tomato
- ½ Cup Shredded cheese

Directions:

1. Let the air fryer preheat to 350°F
2. Lay the pita flat on a plate. Add cheese, slices of tomatoes, and olives.
3. Cook for five minutes at 350°F
4. Take the pizza out of the air fryer.
5. Slice it and enjoy.

Nutrition:

- Calories: 344kcal
- Carbohydrates: 37g
- Protein: 18g
- Fat: 13g

133. Air Fried Cheesy Chicken Omelet

Preparation Time: 5 Minutes
Cooking Time: 18 Minutes
Servings: 2
Ingredients:

- ½ Cup cooked chicken breast, (diced) divided
- 4 Eggs
- 1/4 Tsp. Onion powder, divided
- ½ Tsp. Salt, divided
- 1/4 Tsp. Pepper divided
- 2 Tbsp. Shredded cheese divided
- 1/4 Tsp. Granulated garlic, divided

Directions:

1. Take two ramekins, grease them with olive oil.
2. Add two eggs to each ramekin. Add cheese with seasoning.
3. Blend to combine. Add 1/4 cup of cooked chicken on top.
4. Cook for 14-18 minutes, in the air fryer at 330°F, or until fully cooked.

Nutrition:

- Calories: 185
- Proteins: 20g
- Carbs: 10g
- Fat: 5g

134. 5-Ingredients Air Fryer Lemon Chicken

Preparation Time: 5 Minutes
Cooking Time: 15 Minutes
Servings: 4
Ingredients:

- 1 and ½ cups Whole-wheat crumbs
- 6 Pieces of chicken tenderloins
- Two eggs
- Two half lemons and lemon slices
- Kosher salt to taste

Directions:

1. In a dish, whisk the eggs.
2. In a separate dish, add the breadcrumbs.
3. With egg, coat the chicken and roll in breadcrumbs.
4. Add the breaded chicken to the air fryer.
5. Cook for 14 minutes at 400°F, flip the chicken halfway through.
6. Take out from air fryer and squeeze lemon juice and sprinkle with kosher salt and Serve with lemon slices.

Nutrition:

- Cal: 240
- Fat: 12g
- Net Carbs: 13g
- Protein: 27g

135. Air Fryer Popcorn Chicken

Preparation Time: 10 Minutes
Cooking Time: 20 Minutes
Servings: 2
Ingredients:
For the marinade:

- 8 Cups chicken tenders, cut into bite-size pieces
- ½ Tsp. Freshly ground black pepper
- 2 Cups Almond milk
- 1 Tsp. Salt
- ½ Tsp. Paprika

Dry Mix:

- 3 Tsp. Salt
- 3 Cups Flour
- 2 Tsp. Paprika
- Oil spray
- 2 Tsp. Freshly ground black pepper

Directions:

1. In a bowl, add all marinade ingredients and chicken. Mix well, and put it in a Ziplock bag, and refrigerate for two hours for the minimum, or six hours.

2. In a large bowl, add all the dry ingredients.
3. Coat the marinated chicken to the dry mix. Into the marinade again, then for the second time in the dry mixture.
4. Spray the air fryer basket with olive oil and place the breaded chicken pieces in one single layer. Spray oil over the chicken pieces too.
5. Cook at 370 degrees for 10 minutes, tossing halfway through.
6. Serve immediately with salad greens or dipping sauce.

Nutrition:

- Calories: 340
- Proteins: 20g
- Carbs: 14g
- Fat: 10g

136. Air Fryer Chicken Nuggets

Preparation Time: 15 Minutes
Cooking Time: 15 Minutes
Servings: 4
Ingredients:

- Olive oil spray
- 2 Chicken breasts, skinless boneless, cut into bite pieces
- ½ Tsp. of kosher salt& freshly ground black pepper, to taste 2
- Tablespoons Grated parmesan cheese
- 6 Tablespoons Italian seasoned breadcrumbs (whole wheat)
- 2 Tablespoons whole wheat breadcrumbs
- 2 Teaspoons olive oil
- Panko, optional

Directions:

1. Let the air fryer preheat for 8 minutes to 400°F

2. In a big mixing bowl, add panko, parmesan cheese, and breadcrumbs and mix well.
3. Sprinkle kosher salt and pepper on chicken and olive oil; mix well.
4. Take a few pieces of chicken, dunk them into the breadcrumbs mixture.
5. Put these pieces in an air fryer and spray with olive oil.
6. Cook for 8 minutes, turning halfway through
7. Enjoy with kale chips.

Nutrition:

- Calories: 188kcal
- Carbohydrates: 8g
- Protein: 25g
- Fat: 4.5g

137. Air Fryer Sweet & Sour Chicken

Preparation Time: 5 Minutes
Cooking Time: 10 Minutes
Servings: 2
Ingredients:
Chicken:

- 4 Cups chicken breasts/thighs, cut into one-inch pieces
- 2 Tablespoons cornstarch

Sweet & Sour Sauce:

- 2 Tablespoons cornstarch
- 1 Cup pineapple juice
- 2 Tablespoons water
- Half honey cup
- 1 Tablespoon soy sauce
- 3 Tablespoons rice wine vinegar
- 1/4 Teaspoon ground ginger

Optional:

- 1/4 Cup pineapple chunks
- 3-4 Drops of red food coloring (for traditional orange look)

Directions:

1. Let the air fryer preheat to 400 degrees.
2. Coat the chicken in cornstarch until the chicken is coated completely.
3. Put the chicken in the air fryer and let it cook for 7, 9 minutes. Take it out from the air fryer
4. In the meantime, in a saucepan, add pineapple juice, ginger, honey, soy sauce, and rice wine vinegar and cook. Let it simmer for five minutes.
5. Make cornstarch slurry and add in the sauce. Let it simmer for one minute.
6. Coat cooked chicken pieces and servings with steamed vegetables

Nutrition:

- Cal: 302
- Fat: 8g
- Carbs: 18
- Protein: 22g

138. Low Carb Chicken Tenders

Preparation Time: 10 Minutes
Cooking Time: 20 Minutes
Servings: 3
Ingredients:

- 4 Cups Chicken tenderloins
- 1 Egg
- ½ Cup Superfine Almond Flour
- ½ Cup Powdered Parmesan cheese
- ½ Teaspoon Kosher Sea salt
- 1-Teaspoon freshly ground black pepper
- ½ Teaspoon Cajun seasoning

Directions:

1. On a small plate, pour the beaten egg.
2. Mix all ingredients in a zip lock bag, cheese, almond flour, freshly ground black pepper, kosher salt, and other seasonings.
3. Spray the air fryer with oil spray.
4. To avoid clumpy fingers with breading and egg, use different hands. Dip each tender in egg and then in bread until they are all breaded.
5. Use a fork to place one tender at a time, bring it in the zip lock bag, and shake the bag forcefully, make sure all the tenders are covered in almond mixture
6. Use the fork to take out the tender and place it in your air fryer basket.
7. Spray oil on the tenders.
8. Cook for 12 minutes at 350°F or before 160°F registers within. Raise the temperature to 40°F to shade the surface for 3 minutes.
9. Serve with sauce.

Nutrition:

- Calories: 280
- Proteins 20g
- Carbs: 6g|
- Fat: 10g
- Fiber: 5g

139. Cheesy Cauliflower Tots

Preparation Time: 15 Minutes
Cooking Time: 12 Minutes
Servings: 4
Ingredients:

- 1 Large cauliflower head
- 1 Cup shredded mozzarella cheese
- ½ Cup grated Parmesan cheese
- 1 Large egg
- 1/4 Teaspoon garlic powder
- 1/4 Teaspoon dried parsley
- 1/8 Teaspoon onion powder

Directions:

1. Fill a big pot with 2 cups of water on the stovetop, and insert a steamer in the oven. Put to boil bath.
2. Break the cauliflower into pieces and place them on the steamer box—cover the pot and lid.
3. Let steam the cauliflower for 7 minutes until the fork-tender point. Put in a cheesecloth or clean kitchen towel on the steamer basket and let it cool.
4. Push on the sink to eliminate as much extra humidity as possible. If all of the moisture is not removed, the mixture will be too soft to form into tots.
5. Mash down to a smooth consistency with a blade.
6. In a large mixing bowl, put the cauliflower and add the mozzarella, parmesan, egg, garlic powder, parsley, and onion powder. Remove until well combined. The blend should be smooth but easy to mold.
7. Take two tablespoons of the mixture and roll the mixture into a tot form. Repeat with the rest of the mixture. Put the basket into the air fryer.
8. Set the temperature to 320°F and adjust the timer for 12 minutes.
9. Turn the tots halfway through the period of cooking.
10. Cauliflower tots should be golden when fully cooked. Serve warm.

Nutrition:

- Calories: 181
- Protein 13.5g
- Fiber: 3.0g
- Carbohydrates: 6.6g
- Fat: 9.5g|

Chapter 18. Dessert Recipes

140. Bread Dough and Amaretto Dessert

Preparation Time: 15 Minutes
Cooking Time: 8 Minutes
Servings: 12
Ingredients:

- 1 lb. Bread dough
- 1 Cup sugar
- ½ Cup butter
- 1 Cup heavy cream
- 12 oz. Chocolate chips
- 2 Tbsp. amaretto liqueur

Directions:

1. Turn dough, cut into 20 slices and cut each piece in halves.
2. Put the dough pieces with spray sugar and butter, put this into the air fryer's basket, and cook them at 350°F for 5 minutes. Turn them, cook for 3 minutes still. Move to a platter.
3. Melt the heavy cream in a pan over medium heat, put chocolate chips and turn until they melt.
4. Put in liqueur, turn and move to a bowl.
5. Serve bread dippers with the sauce.

Nutrition:

- Calories: 179
- Total Fat: 18g
- Total carbs: 17g

141. Bread Pudding

Preparation Time: 10 Minutes
Cooking Time: 10 Minutes
Servings: 4
Ingredients:

- 6 Glazed doughnuts
- 1 Cup cherries
- 4 Egg yolks
- 1 and ½ Cups whipping cream
- ½ Cup raisins
- ¼ Cup sugar
- ½ Cup chocolate chips

Directions:

1. Mix in cherries with whipping cream and egg in a bowl, then turn properly.
2. Mix in raisins with chocolate chips, sugar, and doughnuts in a bowl, then stir.
3. Combine the two mixtures, pour into an oiled pan, then into the air fryer, and cook at 310°F for 1 hour.
4. Cool pudding before cutting.
5. Serve.

Nutrition:

- Calories: 456
- Total Fat: 11g
- Total carbs: 6g

142. Wrapped Pears

Preparation Time: 10 Minutes
Cooking Time: 10 Minutes
Servings: 4
Ingredients:

- 4 Puff pastry sheets
- 14 oz. Vanilla custard
- 2 Pears
- 1 Egg
- ½ Tbsp. cinnamon powder
- 2 Tbsp. sugar

Directions:

1. Put wisp pastry slices on a flat surface, add a spoonful of vanilla custard at the center of each, add pear halves and wrap.
2. Combine pears with egg, cinnamon, and spray sugar, put into the air fryer's basket, then cook at 320°F for 15 minutes.
3. Split portions on plates.
4. Serve.

Nutrition:

- Calories: 285
- Total Fat: 14g
- Total carbs: 30g

143. Air Fried Bananas

Preparation Time: 5 Minutes
Cooking Time: 10 Minutes
Servings: 4
Ingredients:

- 3 Tbsp. butter
- 2 Eggs
- 8 Bananas
- ½ Cup corn flour
- 3 Tbsp. cinnamon sugar
- 1 Cup panko

Directions:

1. Heat a pan with the butter over medium heat, put panko, turn and cook for 4 minutes, then move to a bowl.
2. Dredge each in flour, panko, and egg mixture, place in the basket of the air fryer, gratinate with cinnamon sugar, and cook at 280°F for 10 minutes.
3. Serve immediately.

Nutrition:

- Calories: 337
- Total fat: 3g
- Total carbs: 23g

144. Tasty Banana Cake

Preparation Time: 10 Minutes
Cooking Time: 30 Minutes
Servings: 4
Ingredients:

- 1 Tbsp. butter, soft
- 1 Egg
- 1/3 Cup brown sugar
- 2 Tbsp. honey
- 1 Banana
- 1 Cup white flour
- 1 Tbsp. baking powder
- ½ Tbsp. cinnamon powder
- Cooking spray

Directions:

1. Grease the cake pan with cooking spray.
2. Mix in butter with honey, sugar, banana, cinnamon, egg, flour, and baking powder in a bowl, then beat.
3. Put the mix in a cake pan with cooking spray, put into the air fryer, and cook at 350°F for 30 minutes.
4. Allow to cool, then slice it.
5. Serve.

Nutrition:

- Calories: 435
- Total Fat: 7g
- Total carbs: 15g

145. Peanut Butter Fudge

Preparation Time: 10 Minutes
Cooking Time: 10 Minutes
Servings: 20
Ingredients:

- 1/4 Cup almonds, toasted and chopped
- 12 oz. Smooth peanut butter
- 15 Drops liquid stevia
- 3 Tbsp. coconut oil
- 4 Tbsp. coconut cream
- Pinch of salt

Directions:

1. Line a baking tray with parchment paper.
2. Melt coconut oil in a pan over low heat. Add peanut butter, coconut cream, stevia, and salt to a saucepan. Stir well.
3. Pour fudge mixture into the prepared baking tray and sprinkle chopped almonds on top.
4. Place the tray in the refrigerator for 1 hour or until set.
5. Slice and serve.

Nutrition:

- Calories: 131
- Fat: 12g
- Carbs: 4g
- Sugar: 2g
- Protein: 5g
- Cholesterol: 0mg

146. Cocoa Cake

Preparation Time: 5 Minutes
Cooking Time: 17 Minutes
Servings: 6
Ingredients:

- 4 oz. Butter

- 3 Eggs
- 3 oz. Sugar
- 1 Tbsp. cocoa powder
- 3 oz. Flour
- ½ Tbsp. lemon juice

Directions:

1. Mix in 1 tablespoon butter with cocoa powder in a bowl and beat.
2. Mix in the rest of the butter with eggs, flour, sugar, and lemon juice in another bowl, blend properly and move the half into a cake pan
3. Put half of the cocoa blend, spread, add the rest of the butter layer, and crest with remaining cocoa.
4. Put into the air fryer and cook at 360° F for 17 minutes.
5. Allow it to cool before slicing.
6. Serve.

Nutrition:

- Calories: 221
- Total Fat: 5g
- Total carbs: 12g

147. Avocado Pudding

Preparation Time: 20 Minutes
Cooking Time: 0 Minutes
Servings: 8
Ingredients:

- 2 Ripe avocados, pitted and cut into pieces
- 1 Tbsp. fresh lime juice
- 14 oz. Can coconut milk
- 2 Tsp. liquid stevia
- 2 Tsp. vanilla

Directions:

1. Inside the blender, add all ingredients and blend until smooth.
2. Serve immediately and enjoy.

Nutrition:

- Calories: 317
- Fat: 30g
- Carbs: 9g
- Sugar: 0.5g
- Protein: 3g
- Cholesterol: 0mg

148. Bounty Bars

Preparation Time: 20 Minutes
Cooking Time: 0 Minutes
Servings: 12
Ingredients:

- 1 Cup coconut cream
- 3 Cups shredded unsweetened coconut
- 1/4 Cup extra virgin coconut oil
- ½ Teaspoon vanilla powder
- 1/4 Cup powdered erythritol
- 1 ½ oz. Cocoa butter
- 5 oz. Dark chocolate

Directions:

1. Heat the oven at 350°F and toast the coconut in it for 5-6 minutes. Remove from the oven once toasted and set aside to cool.
2. Take a bowl of medium size and add coconut oil, coconut cream, vanilla, erythritol, and shredded coconut. Mix the ingredients well to prepare a smooth mixture.
3. Make 12 bars of equal size with the help of your hands from the prepared mixture and adjust in the tray lined with parchment paper.
4. Place the tray in the fridge for around one hour and, in the meantime, put the cocoa butter and dark chocolate in a glass bowl.
5. Heat a cup of water in a saucepan over medium heat and place the bowl over it to melt the cocoa butter and the dark chocolate.
6. Remove from the heat once melted properly, mix well until blended, and set it aside to cool.
7. Take the coconut bars and coat them with dark chocolate mixture one by one using a wooden stick. Adjust on the tray lined with parchment paper and drizzle the remaining mixture over them.
8. Refrigerate for around one hour before you serve the delicious bounty bars.

Nutrition:

- Calories: 230
- Fat: 25g
- Carbohydrates: 5g
- Protein: 32g

149. Simple Cheesecake

Preparation Time: 10 Minutes
Cooking Time: 15 Minutes
Servings: 15
Ingredients:

- 1 lb. Cream cheese
- ½ Tbsp. vanilla extract
- 2 Eggs
- 4 Tbsp. sugar
- 1 Cup graham crackers
- 2 Tbsp. butter

Directions:

1. Mix in butter with crackers in a bowl.
2. Compress crackers blend to the bottom of a cake pan, put into the air fryer, and cook at 350°F for 4 minutes.
3. Mix cream cheese with sugar, vanilla, egg in a bowl and beat properly.
4. Sprinkle filling on crackers crust and cook the cheesecake in the air fryer at 310°F for 15 minutes.
5. Keep the cake in the fridge for 3 hours, slice.
6. Serve.

Nutrition:

- Calories: 257
- Total Fat: 18g
- Total carbs: 22g

150. Chocolate Almond Butter Brownie

Preparation Time: 10 Minutes
Cooking Time: 16 Minutes
Servings: 4
Ingredients:

- 1 Cup bananas, overripe
- ½ Cup almond butter, melted
- 1 Scoop protein powder
- 2 Tbsp. unsweetened cocoa powder

Directions:

1. Preheat the air fryer to 325°F. Grease the air fryer baking pan and set it aside.
2. Blend all ingredients in a blender until smooth.
3. Pour the batter into the prepared pan and place it in the air fryer basket to cook for 16 minutes.
4. Serve and enjoy.

Nutrition:

- Calories: 82
- Fat: 2g
- Carbs: 11g
- Sugar: 5g
- Protein: 7g
- Cholesterol: 16mg

151. Almond Butter Fudge

Preparation Time: 10 Minutes
Cooking Time: 10 Minutes
Servings: 18
Ingredients:

- 3/4 Cup creamy almond butter
- 1 ½ Cups unsweetened chocolate chips

Directions:

1. Line 8x4-inch pan with parchment paper and set aside.
2. Add chocolate chips and almond butter into the double boiler and cook over medium heat until the chocolate-butter mixture is melted. Stir well.
3. Place the mixture into the prepared pan and place in the freezer until set.
4. Slice and serve.

Nutrition:

- Calories: 197
- Fat: 16g
- Carbs: 7g
- Sugar: 1g
- Protein: 4g
- Cholesterol: 0mg

152. Apple Bread

Preparation Time: 5 Minutes
Cooking Time: 40 Minutes
Servings: 6
Ingredients:

- 3 Cups apples
- 1 Cup sugar
- 1 Tbsp. vanilla
- 2 Eggs
- 1 Tbsp. apple pie spice
- 2 Cups white flour
- 1 Tbsp. baking powder
- 1 Butter stick
- 1 Cup water

Directions:

1. Mix the eggs with one butter stick, sugar, vanilla, and apple pie spice, then turn using a mixer.
2. Put apples and turn properly.
3. Mix baking powder with flour in another bowl and turn.
4. Blend the two mixtures, turn and move it to a springform pan.
5. Put the pan into the air fryer and cook at 320°F for 40 minutes
6. Slice.
7. Serve.

Nutrition:

- Calories: 401
- Total Fat: 9g
- Total carbs: 29g

153. Banana Bread

Preparation Time: 5 Minutes
Cooking Time: 40 Minutes
Servings: 6
Ingredients:

- ¾ Cup sugar
- 1/3 Cup butter
- 1 Tbsp. vanilla extract
- 1 Egg
- 2 Bananas
- 1 Tbsp. baking powder
- 1 and ½ Cups flour
- ½ Tbsp. baking soda
- 1/3 Cup milk
- 1 and ½ Tbsp. cream of tartar
- Cooking spray

Directions:

1. Mix the milk with cream of tartar, vanilla, egg, sugar, bananas, and butter in a bowl, then mix all.
2. Mix in flour with baking soda and baking powder.
3. Blend the two mixtures, turn properly, move into an oiled pan with cooking spray, put into the air fryer, and cook at 320°F for 40 minutes.
4. Remove the bread, allow to cool, slice.
5. Serve.

Nutrition:

- Calories: 540
- Total Fat: 16g
- Total carbs: 28g

154. Mini Lava Cakes

Preparation Time: 5 Minutes
Cooking Time: 20 Minutes
Servings: 3
Ingredients:

- 1 Egg
- 4 Tbsp. sugar
- 2 Tbsp. olive oil
- 4 Tbsp. milk
- 4 Tbsp. flour
- 1 Tbsp. cocoa powder
- ½ Tbsp. baking powder
- ½ Tbsp. orange zest
- A pinch of salt

Directions:

1. Mix in egg with sugar, flour, salt, oil, milk, orange zest, baking powder, and cocoa powder, turn properly. Move it to oiled ramekins.
2. Put ramekins in the air fryer and cook at 320°F for 20 minutes.
3. Serve warm.

Nutrition:

- Calories: 329
- Total Fat: 8.5g
- Total carbs: 12.4g

155. Ricotta Ramekins

Preparation Time: 10 Minutes
Cooking Time: 1 Hour
Servings: 4
Ingredients:

- 6 Eggs, whisked
- 1 and ½ Pounds ricotta cheese, soft
- ½ Pound stevia
- 1 Teaspoon vanilla extract
- ½ Teaspoon baking powder
- Cooking spray

Directions:

1. In a bowl, mix the eggs with the ricotta and the other ingredients except for the cooking spray and whisk well.
2. Grease 4 ramekins with the cooking spray, pour the ricotta cream in each and bake at 360 degrees F for 1 hour.
3. Serve cold.

Nutrition:

- Calories: 180
- Fat: 5.3
- Fiber: 5.4
- Carbs: 11.5
- Protein: 4

156. Strawberry Sorbet

Preparation Time: 15 Minutes
Cooking Time: 10 Minutes
Servings: 6
Ingredients:

- 1 Cup strawberries, chopped
- 1 Tablespoon of liquid honey
- 2 Tablespoons water
- 1 Tablespoon lemon juice

Directions:

1. Preheat the water and liquid honey until you get a homogenous liquid.
2. Blend the strawberries until smooth and combine them with the honey liquid and lemon juice.
3. Transfer the strawberry mixture to the ice cream maker and churn it for 20 minutes or until the sorbet is thick.
4. Scoop the cooked sorbet in the ice cream cups.

Nutrition:

- Calories: 30
- Fat: 0.4g
- Fiber: 1.4g
- Carbs: 14.9g
- Protein: 0.9g

157. Crispy Apples

Preparation Time: 10 Minutes
Cooking Time: 10 Minutes
Servings: 4
Ingredients:

- 2 Tbsp. cinnamon powder
- 5 Apples
- ½ Tbsp. nutmeg powder
- 1 Tbsp. maple syrup
- ½ Cup water
- 4 Tbsp. butter
- ¼ Cup flour
- ¾ Cup oats
- ¼ Cup brown sugar

Directions:

1. Get the apples in a pan, put in nutmeg, maple syrup, cinnamon, and water.
2. Mix in butter with flour, sugar, salt, and oat, turn, put a spoonful of the blend over apples, get into the air fryer and cook at 350°F for 10 minutes.
3. Serve while warm.

Nutrition:

- Calories: 387
- Total Fat: 5.6g
- Total carbs: 12.4g

158. Cocoa Cookies

Preparation Time: 10 Minutes
Cooking Time: 14 Minutes
Servings: 12
Ingredients:

- 6 oz. Coconut oil
- 6 Eggs
- 3 oz. Cocoa powder
- 2 Tbsp. vanilla
- ½ Tbsp. baking powder
- 4 oz. Cream cheese
- 5 Tbsp. sugar

Directions:

1. Mix the eggs with sugar, coconut oil, baking powder, cocoa powder, cream cheese, vanilla in a blender, then sway and turn using a mixer.
2. Get it into a lined baking dish and put it into the fryer at 320°F, and bake for 14 minutes.
3. Split cookie sheet into rectangles.
4. Serve.

Nutrition:

- Calories: 149
- Total Fat: 2.4g
- Total carbs: 27.2g

159. Cinnamon Pears

Preparation Time: 2 Hours
Cooking Time: 0 Minutes
Servings: 6
Ingredients:

- 2 Pears
- 1 Teaspoon ground cinnamon
- 1 Tablespoon Erythritol
- 1 Teaspoon liquid stevia
- 4 Teaspoons butter

Directions:

1. Cut the pears on the halves.
2. Then scoop the seeds from the pears with the help of the scooper.
3. In a shallow bowl, mix up together Erythritol and ground cinnamon.
4. Sprinkle every pear half with cinnamon mixture and drizzle with liquid stevia.
5. Then add butter and wrap in the foil.
6. Bake the pears for 25 minutes at 365°F.
7. Then remove the pears from the foil and transfer them to the serving plates.

Nutrition:

- Calories: 96
- Fat: 4.4g
- Fiber: 1.4g
- Carbs: 3.9g
- Protein: 0.9g

160. Cherry Compote

Preparation Time: 2 Hours
Cooking Time: 0 Minutes
Servings: 6
Ingredients:

- 2 Peaches, pitted, halved
- 1 Cup cherries, pitted
- ½ Cup grape juice
- ½ Cup strawberries
- 1 Tablespoon liquid honey
- 1 Teaspoon vanilla extract
- 1 Teaspoon ground cinnamon

Directions:

1. Pour grape juice into the saucepan.
2. Add vanilla extract and ground cinnamon. Bring the liquid to a boil.
3. After this, put peaches, cherries, and strawberries in the hot grape juice and bring them to a boil.
4. Remove the mixture from heat, add liquid honey, and close the lid.
5. Let the compote rest for 20 minutes.
6. Carefully mix up the compote and transfer it to the serving plate.

Nutrition:

- Calories: 80
- Fat: 0.4g
- Fiber: 2.4g
- Carbs: 19.9g
- Protein: 0.9g

CPSIA information can be obtained
at www.ICGtesting.com
Printed in the USA
LVHW031026010621
689027LV00012B/1669